NUTRITION AND HEALTIIY AGING IN THE COMMUNITY

WORKSHOP SUMMARY

W9-BBZ-047

Sheila Moats and Julia Hoglund, *Rapporteurs*

Food and Nutrition Board

INSTITUTE OF MEDICINE
OF THE NATIONAL ACADEMIES

THE NATIONAL ACADEMIES PRESS
Washington, D.C.
www.nap.edu

THE NATIONAL ACADEMIES PRESS   500 Fifth Street, NW   Washington, DC 20001

NOTICE: The project that is the subject of this report was approved by the Governing Board of the National Research Council, whose members are drawn from the councils of the National Academy of Sciences, the National Academy of Engineering, and the Institute of Medicine.

This study was supported by Contract No. N01-OD-4-2139, Task Order No. 235, between the National Academy of Sciences and the National Institutes of Health (Division of Nutrition Research Coordination and Office of Dietary Supplements) and by Contract No. HHSP233201100557P from the U.S. Department of Health and Human Services (Administration on Aging), and grants from Abbott Laboratories, the Meals On Wheels Association of America, and the Meals On Wheels Research Foundation. Any opinions, findings, conclusions, or recommendations expressed in this publication are those of the author(s) and do not necessarily reflect the view of the organizations or agencies that provided support for this project.

International Standard Book Number-13:   978-0-309-25310-9
International Standard Book Number-10:   0-309-25310-1

Additional copies of this report are available from the National Academies Press, 500 Fifth Street, NW, Keck 360, Washington, DC 20001; (800) 624-6242 or (202) 334-3313; http://www.nap.edu.

For more information about the Institute of Medicine, visit the IOM home page at: www.iom.edu.

The serpent has been a symbol of long life, healing, and knowledge among almost all cultures and religions since the beginning of recorded history. The serpent adopted as a logotype by the Institute of Medicine is a relief carving from ancient Greece, now held by the Staatliche Museen in Berlin.

Suggested citation: IOM (Institute of Medicine). 2012. *Nutrition and Healthy Aging in the Community: Workshop Summary.* Washington, DC: The National Academies Press.

*"Knowing is not enough; we must apply.
Willing is not enough; we must do."*
—Goethe

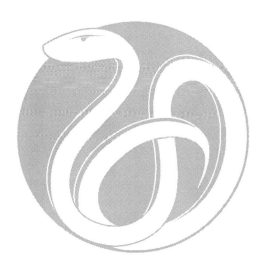

INSTITUTE OF MEDICINE
OF THE NATIONAL ACADEMIES

Advising the Nation. Improving Health.

THE NATIONAL ACADEMIES
Advisers to the Nation on Science, Engineering, and Medicine

The **National Academy of Sciences** is a private, nonprofit, self-perpetuating society of distinguished scholars engaged in scientific and engineering research, dedicated to the furtherance of science and technology and to their use for the general welfare. Upon the authority of the charter granted to it by the Congress in 1863, the Academy has a mandate that requires it to advise the federal government on scientific and technical matters. Dr. Ralph J. Cicerone is president of the National Academy of Sciences.

The **National Academy of Engineering** was established in 1964, under the charter of the National Academy of Sciences, as a parallel organization of outstanding engineers. It is autonomous in its administration and in the selection of its members, sharing with the National Academy of Sciences the responsibility for advising the federal government. The National Academy of Engineering also sponsors engineering programs aimed at meeting national needs, encourages education and research, and recognizes the superior achievements of engineers. Dr. Charles M. Vest is president of the National Academy of Engineering.

The **Institute of Medicine** was established in 1970 by the National Academy of Sciences to secure the services of eminent members of appropriate professions in the examination of policy matters pertaining to the health of the public. The Institute acts under the responsibility given to the National Academy of Sciences by its congressional charter to be an adviser to the federal government and, upon its own initiative, to identify issues of medical care, research, and education. Dr. Harvey V. Fineberg is president of the Institute of Medicine.

The **National Research Council** was organized by the National Academy of Sciences in 1916 to associate the broad community of science and technology with the Academy's purposes of furthering knowledge and advising the federal government. Functioning in accordance with general policies determined by the Academy, the Council has become the principal operating agency of both the National Academy of Sciences and the National Academy of Engineering in providing services to the government, the public, and the scientific and engineering communities. The Council is administered jointly by both Academies and the Institute of Medicine. Dr. Ralph J. Cicerone and Dr. Charles M. Vest are chair and vice chair, respectively, of the National Research Council.

www.national-academies.org

PLANNING COMMITTEE ON NUTRITION AND HEALTHY AGING IN THE COMMUNITY: A WORKSHOP*

GORDON L. JENSEN (*Chair*), Professor and Head, Department of
    Nutritional Sciences, Pennsylvania State University, University Park
CONNIE W. BALES, Professor of Medicine, Division of Geriatrics, Duke
    University, NC and the Geriatric Research, Education, and Clinical
    Center, Durham VA Medical Center, NC
ELIZABETH B. LANDON, Vice President, Community Services,
    CareLink, North Little Rock, AR
JULIE L. LOCHER, Associate Professor of Medicine, Division of
    Gerontology, Geriatrics, and Palliative Care, University of Alabama,
    Birmingham
DOUGLAS PADDON-JONES, Associate Professor, Department
    of Nutrition and Metabolism, School of Health Professionals,
    Department of Internal Medicine, The University of Texas Medical
    Branch, Galveston
NADINE R. SAHYOUN, Associate Professor, Department of Nutrition
    and Food Science, University of Maryland, College Park
NANCY S. WELLMAN, Adjunct Professor, Friedman School of Nutrition
    Science and Policy, Tufts University, Boston, MA

IOM Staff

SHEILA MOATS, Study Director
JULIA HOGLUND, Research Associate
ALLISON BERGER, Senior Program Assistant
ANTON L. BANDY, Financial Associate
GERALDINE KENNEDO, Administrative Assistant
LINDA D. MEYERS, Director, Food and Nutrition Board

---

*Institute of Medicine planning committees are solely responsible for organizing the workshop, identifying topics, and choosing speakers. The responsibility for the published workshop summary rests with the workshop rapporteur and the institution.

Reviewers

This report has been reviewed in draft form by individuals chosen for their diverse perspectives and technical expertise, in accordance with procedures approved by the National Research Council's Report Review Committee. The purpose of this independent review is to provide candid and critical comments that will assist the institution in making its published report as sound as possible and to ensure that the report meets institutional standards for objectivity, evidence, and responsiveness to the study charge. The review comments and draft manuscript remain confidential to protect the integrity of the process. We wish to thank the following individuals for their review of this report:

Rose Ann DiMaria-Ghalili, Doctoral Nursing Department and
    Nutrition Sciences Department, Drexel University, Philadelphia, PA
Denise K. Houston, Department of Internal Medicine, Section on
    Gerontology and Geriatric Medicine, Wake Forest School of
    Medicine, Winston-Salem, NC
Gordon Jensen, Department of Nutritional Sciences, Pennsylvania
    State University, University Park
Nadine R. Sahyoun, Department of Nutrition and Food Sciences,
    University of Maryland, College Park
Dennis T. Villareal, New Mexico VA Health Care System,
    Albuquerque

Although the reviewers listed above have provided many constructive comments and suggestions, they did not see the final draft of the report before its release. The review of this report was overseen by **Hugh H. Tilson,** University of North Carolina at Chapel Hill. Appointed by the Institute of Medicine, he was responsible for making certain that an independent examination of this report was carried out in accordance with institutional procedures and that all review comments were carefully considered. Responsibility for the final content of this report rests entirely with the authors and the institution.

Contents

Overview[1]

The U.S. population of older adults[2] is predicted to grow rapidly as baby boomers (those born between 1946 and 1964) begin to reach 65 years of age. Simultaneously, advancements in medical care and improved awareness of healthy lifestyles have led to longer life expectancies. The Census Bureau projects that the population of Americans 65 years of age and older will rise from approximately 40 million in 2010 to 55 million in 2020, a 36 percent increase (AoA, 2010). Furthermore, older adults are choosing to live independently in the community setting rather than residing in an institutional environment. This increase in the older population will result in a surge in the demand for delivery of services and create new challenges for older people, their caregivers, and nutrition and social services professionals who seek to ensure the availability of services to this population.

The types of services needed by this population are shifting due to changes in their health issues. Older adults have historically been viewed as underweight and frail; however, over the past decade there has been an increase in the number of obese older persons. Obesity in older adults is not only associated with medical comorbidities such as diabetes; it is also

---

[1]The planning committee's role was limited to planning the workshop, and the workshop summary has been prepared by the workshop rapporteurs as a factual summary of what occurred at the workshop. Statements, recommendations, and opinions expressed are those of individual presenters and participants, and are not necessarily endorsed or verified by the Institute of Medicine, and they should not be construed as reflecting any group consensus.

[2]According to the World Health Organization, "most developed world countries have accepted the chronological age of 65 years as a definition of . . . older person." http://www. who.int/healthinfo/survey/ageingdefnolder/en/index.html.

1

a major risk factor for functional decline and homebound status (Jensen et al., 2006). The baby boomers have a greater prevalence of obesity than any of their historic counterparts, and projections forecast an aging population with even greater chronic disease burden and disability.

Nutrition is a key component to promoting healthy and functional living among older adults. The 2000 Institute of Medicine (IOM) report *The Role of Nutrition in Maintaining Health in the Nation's Elderly: Evaluating Coverage of Nutrition Services for the Medicare Population* highlighted priorities for enhanced coverage and coordination of nutrition services in the community setting. Little progress has been made toward meeting those priorities during the decade since the report was published. Nutrition services are fragmented and poorly integrated with other services. In addition, coverage and reimbursement continue to have serious limitations, thus increasing the possibility that older adults requiring nutrition services will fall through gaps in this tenuous service net.

In light of the increasing numbers of older adults choosing to live independently rather than in nursing homes, and the important role nutrition can play in healthy aging, the IOM convened a public workshop to illuminate issues related to community-based delivery of nutrition services for older adults and to identify nutrition interventions and model programs which promote (1) successful transitions from acute, subacute, and chronic care to home and (2) health and independent living in the community, as well as to highlight needed research priorities. It is envisioned that the workshop will improve awareness and understanding of technical and policy issues related to nutrition needs of older adults in community settings by fostering increased dialogue among health, nutrition, and social services policy makers and researchers. This foundation will facilitate better informed and more effective plans and decisions by government and non-government policy makers, implementing agencies, and others informed by the workshop and this summary.

The workshop, sponsored by the Department of Health and Human Services Administration on Aging, the National Institutes of Health Division of Nutrition Research Coordination and Office of Dietary Supplements, the Meals On Wheels Association of America, the Meals On Wheels Research Foundation, and Abbott Nutrition, was held on October 5–6, 2011, in Washington, DC. The workshop agenda appears in Appendix A. The IOM-appointed workshop planning committee was chaired by Dr. Gordon L. Jensen of The Pennsylvania State University, who also served as the overall moderator for the workshop. Each member of the planning committee, listed in the front matter of this report, contributed to the substance of the agenda and moderated the presentations and discussions for the five sessions.

This report is a summary of the presentations and discussions prepared from the workshop transcript and slides. The report is organized according to the chronological order of the proceedings. Chapter 1 provides an introduction; a summary of the keynote address on the demographics of the aging population and resources available to them; and a case study of an older adult who, with the assistance of nutrition and other services, transi-￼ ￼ ￼ ￼ ￼ ￼ ￼. Chapter 2 examines nutrition-related issues of concern experienced by older adults in the community including nutrition screening, food insecurity, sarcopenic obesity, dietary patterns for older adults, and economic issues. Chapter 3 explores transitional care as individuals move from acute, subacute, or chronic care settings to the community, and Chapter 4 provides models of transitional care in the community. Chapter 5 provides examples of successful intervention models in the community setting, and Chapter 6 covers the discussion of research gaps in knowledge about nutrition interventions and services for older adults in the community. This workshop summary highlights issues and presents recommendations made by individual speakers, but it does not represent consensus recommendations of the workshop.

Appendixes at the end of the report provide additional information. As mentioned above, the workshop agenda is reproduced in Appendix A. The workshop planning committee and speakers' biographical sketches appear in Appendix B, the names and affiliations of workshop attendees are compiled in Appendix C, and a guide to the acronyms and abbreviations used throughout the report is provided in Appendix D.

REFERENCES

AoA (Administration on Aging, Department of Health and Human Services). 2010. *A Profile of Older Americans: 2010.* http://www.aoa.gov/AoARoot/Aging_StatisticsProfile/2010/docs/2010profile.pdf (accessed October 18, 2011).

Jensen, G. L., H. J. Silver, M.-A. Roy, E. Callahan, C. Still, and W. Dupont. 2006. Obesity is a risk factor for reporting homebound status among community-dwelling older persons. *Obesity* 14(3):509–517.

1

Introduction

WELCOME, INTRODUCTION, AND PURPOSE

Presenter: Gordon L. Jensen

Gordon Jensen opened the workshop by welcoming participants and sharing background on the development of the workshop. More than a decade ago Jensen was part of an Institute of Medicine committee that examined nutrition services for Medicare beneficiaries. In that report, the committee identified impressive gaps in coverage and knowledge related to nutrition services in the community setting for older persons. Recognizing little progress in filling those gaps, in 2008 the Food and Nutrition Board (FNB) proposed a workshop to address nutrition services in the community setting.

Jensen thanked the planning committee for developing the workshop agenda in a short time frame, as well as the workshop sponsors, and the FNB. Specifically, he acknowledged the sponsors:

- National Institutes of Health (NIH) Division of Nutrition Research Coordination
- NIH Office of Dietary Supplements
- Department of Health and Human Services Administration on Aging
- Meals On Wheels Association of America
- Meals On Wheels Research Foundation
- Abbott Nutrition

Jensen then introduced Edwin Walker, Deputy Assistant Secretary for Program Operations at the Department of Health and Human Services Administration on Aging, who gave the keynote address.

THE AGING LANDSCAPE IN THE COMMUNITY SETTING

Presenter: Edwin L. Walker

Walker began by bringing greetings on behalf of the Administration on Aging (AoA) and the Assistant Secretary for Aging, Kathy Greenlee. He also thanked the audience for bringing attention to critical issues related to nutrition.

Walker described AoA as a federal agency that, in statute, is charged with advocating and "somewhat intruding" into the policy making of other federal agencies, state agencies, or any entity whose activities may impact the life of an older person. Walker said that the mission of AoA (Box 1-1) is consistent with basic American values.

Because the AoA knows that older people prefer to reside at home rather than in institutional settings such as nursing homes, its network provides supports that enable older adults to maintain their health and independence in the community for as long as possible. Walker noted that support is also included for family caregivers of older adults.

History of the Older Americans Act

> *Every state and every community can now move toward a coordinated program of services and opportunities for our older citizens.*
>
> —President Lyndon B. Johnson, July 1965

The Older Americans Act (OAA) was created in 1965 and signed into law 15 days before Medicare and Medicaid as one part of a three-part strategy in President Johnson's "War on Poverty." Medicare provided healthcare for older adults and people with disabilities, while Medicaid provided health care and supports for indigent individuals. Walker explained that the OAA was part of a plan that included Medicare and Medicaid and, although not designed as such, evolved into provision of long-term care in nursing homes. In the 1980s, Medicaid officials acknowledged that people did not want care in nursing homes by creating home- and community-based service waivers to support the provision of care in individuals' homes.

Medicare and Medicaid are referred to as entitlements since they are

---

BOX 1-1
Administration on Aging's Mission

To help elderly individuals maintain their dignity and independence in their homes and communities through comprehensive, coordinated, and cost-effective systems of long-term care, and livable communities across the United States.

SOURCE: AoA, 2011a.

---

funded through mandatory appropriations, and, as a result, eligibility entitles a person to receive all benefits provided under the program. In contrast, the OAA is a discretionary program funded through annual appropriations, and individual need is assessed. It is designed to be a complement to the entitlements. OAA was planned to assist older adults in a way that would maintain their dignity and avoid their perception of the stigma associated with participating in a welfare program. It was structured to function as a partnership with state and local governments, nongovernmental entities, and, most importantly, consumers. Walker explained that the success of the program can be attributed to older adults' real sense of ownership of the program. Often at the local level it is not viewed as a federal program, but as a local community program.

AoA programs were always planned to be two-pronged, as stated in President Johnson's quote. One goal is to provide services that respond to individual needs and the second is to acknowledge that opportunities need to be developed for older adults in recognition of their wealth of knowledge and ability to contribute to society. AoA programs are available to anyone over the age of 60 years, but they are targeted to those in greatest social and economic need with particular attention to low-income minority older individuals, older individuals who reside in rural communities, limited English–speaking individuals, and those who are at risk of nursing home admission.

Demographics

Currently, about one in eight individuals in this country (13 percent) is an older American (U.S. Census Bureau, 2011) and, based on the current life expectancy rate, he or she can expect to live on average another 18.6 years (NCHS, 2011). Thirty percent of these older Americans live alone; since older women outnumber older men, 50 percent of older women live alone. Twenty percent of these older Americans are minorities (AoA, 2010). The numbers continue to grow rapidly. In fact, 9,000 baby boomers turn 65 years old every day. In 4 years the population of people over the age of 60 years will increase by 15 percent, from 57 million to 65.7 million. During this period the number of people with severe disabilities who are at greatest risk for nursing home admission and for Medicaid eligibility will increase by more than 13 percent. Similar patterns are seen in demographics on the global level. It is predicted that by 2045 the population of older people in the world will be higher than that of children for the first time in history (United Nations Department of Economic and Social Affairs, Population Division, 2010).

Characteristics of the older population include high levels of multiple chronic conditions, hospital admissions and readmissions, and emergency room usage. Walker indicated that statistics show participants in AoA programs take 10 or more prescription drugs on a daily basis. These older adults also have extensive limitations in terms of their activities of daily living and instrumental activities of daily living, resulting in low functional levels and, therefore, requiring physical assistance.

The Aging Network

The Aging Network, depicted in Figure 1-1 and created by the OAA, has evolved into this country's infrastructure for home- and community-based services. Part of the mission is to coordinate with all of the other funding streams and organizations that touch the lives of older people. As a result of the OAA about 11 million older adults are served annually, that is, one in five older adults in this country (HHS, 2012). They are provided with low-cost nonmedical community-based services and interventions. Programs are moving toward evidence-based interventions in order to have the greatest effect on improving outcomes in an individual's health and well-being.

The AoA is at the top of the pyramid in Figure 1-1. AoA is a very small federal agency because its strength is at the local community level. It does not provide a prescriptive set of guidelines, but it establishes basic principles describing goals to be achieved at the local level. AoA relates in a partnership manner with states and tribes, who in turn use their sovereign relationship with regional and local service areas to designate area agencies to assess what is needed in their own communities and ensure that the funds are spent in ways that are responsive to those needs.

Contracts are established with more than 20,000 local service providers, including nonprofit, faith-based, and nongovernmental entities, which Walker referred to as AoA's "real strength." These local service providers use the resources of more than 500,000 volunteers, often older people themselves who have a sense of ownership in the program and want to give back their time and resources to ensure the continuation of

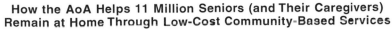

How the AoA Helps 11 Million Seniors (and Their Caregivers)
Remain at Home Through Low-Cost Community-Based Services

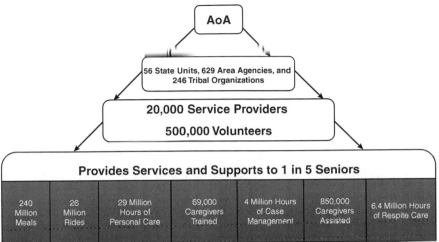

FIGURE 1-1 The Aging Network.
SOURCE: Walker, 2011.

services for others in need. Some of these services are listed at the bottom
of the pyramid (Figure 1 1). Walker noted that consumers provide input
into the design of these programs at every level—local, regional, and state.

Walker noted it takes an array of services provided by the Aging Network in the community, collaborating to achieve the mission of keeping
an individual at home. These are cost-effective services and programs; the
extent of contributions made at the state and local levels and by participants themselves are so significant that, for every federal dollar spent, the
program generates, on average, another $3.

Many of the current programs evolved from pilot projects or demon-
strations, including the nutrition program, the concept of a regional area
agency on aging, and the concept of a community-based service delivery
network. After demonstrating that these programs were successful models
that adequately responded to individuals' needs, they became permanent
programs and features of the OAA Aging Network.

Person-Centered Approach

The OAA Aging Network has always focused on a person-centered
approach to the delivery of services, creating a system and a culture that

coordinates all available resources to serve the needs of an individual. AoA collaborates with other agencies and health care systems to link services, seizing opportunities to more efficiently serve individuals.

Examples of such collaboration include working with the Centers for Medicare & Medicaid Services in the health care sector, and encouraging the local network to partner with hospitals and other health care systems to provide a more holistic approach and explore implementation of a person-centered approach. In the area of public health, AoA is partnering with the Health Resources and Services Administration to connect with community health centers and federally qualified health clinics. Other collaborative efforts include working with the Centers for Disease Control and Prevention on prevention issues; with NIH on the translation of research into practice at the local level; with the Department of Housing and Urban Development on coordination of services for people in public housing facilities; and with the Department of Transportation (DOT) to coordinate transportation for older adults through DOT's United We Ride initiative. On an individual basis, AoA provides assistance and information that will help older adults to age in place. This includes providing information on mortgages, pensions, public and private benefits, and protective and legal services.

Walker drew attention to the partnership developed with the Veterans Administration (VA). Rather than creating its own home- and community-based system, the VA approached AoA and now purchases services for veterans from the Aging Network. Further information on this collaborative effort was presented by Daniel Schoeps and Lori Gerhard later in the workshop (see Chapter 4).

Nutrition Services and Food Insecurity

AoA's nutrition program is the organization's largest health program, providing meals and assistance in preparing meals. There are three primary nutrition programs: Congregate Nutrition Services (CN), Home-Delivered Nutrition Services (HDN), and a Nutrition Services Incentive Program. Walker reported the costs of these programs in fiscal year (FY) 2010:

- Total federal, state, and local expenditures: $1.4 billion
- Annual expenditure per person: $370 (CN), $895 (HDN)
- Expenditures per meal: $6.64 (CN), $5.34 (HDN)

Also in FY 2010, HDN provided approximately 145 million meals to more than 880,000 older adults and CN provided over 96.4 million meals to more than 1.7 million older adults in a variety of community settings (HHS, 2012). Adequate nutrition is necessary for health, functionality, and the ability to remain at home in the community. Walker reported 90 percent of AoA clients have multiple chronic conditions, which can be ameliorated through proper nutrition. Furthermore, 35 percent of older adults receiving home-delivered meals are unable to perform three or more activities of daily living, while 69 percent are unable to perform three or more instrumental activities of daily living, putting them at risk for emergency room visits, hospital readmissions, and nursing home admissions.

Sixty-three percent of HDN clients and 58 percent of CN clients report that the one meal provided under these programs is half or more of their food intake for the day (AoA, 2011b). Researchers estimate that food-insecure older adults are so functionally impaired it is as if they are chronologically 14 years older (e.g., a 65-year-old food-insecure individual is like a 79-year-old chronologically) (Ziliak and Gundersen, 2011). Walker reported that malnourishment declines upon receiving HDN meals, as indicated by the fact that the number of HDN participants eating fewer than two meals per day decreased by 57 percent. Yet, despite receiving five meals per week, 24 percent of HDN participants and 13 percent of CN participants did not have enough money to buy food for the remaining meals in that week. Seventeen percent of HDN participants indicate that they have to choose between purchasing food and purchasing their medications, and 15 percent of the HDN participants have to choose between paying for food, rent, and utilities (AoA, 2011b). A more in-depth presentation on food insecurity in older adults was presented by James Ziliak (see Chapter 2.)

Closing Remarks

Walker concluded that the work of AoA is an ongoing process. Programs continue to be developed or refined to meet the ever-increasing and changing needs of the older population. More culturally competent, culturally sensitive programs need to be incorporated, as well as more flexible programs that adapt to the needs of the people. "We need to be in the mode of ever evolving, ever changing, ever improving to meet the needs of the current and the future seniors, as well as their caregivers," said Walker. He expressed the belief that the workshop will significantly aid the future design of AoA so it can meet those needs.

DISCUSSION

Moderator: Gordon L. Jensen

During the discussion, points raised by participants centered on reaching older adults in need. Robert Miller noted that AoA is reaching one in five older adults and asked if Walker thought that the remaining four people also need assistance. The Aging Network is responsible for and, Walker believes, is doing well at targeting those most at risk. For those that are not receiving services from AoA, there are a variety of reasons. It may be due to a lack of awareness on the part of either AoA or the older adult in need, while others may receive nonfederally funded assistance or assistance from their families. Walker noted that a comprehensive assessment is done to determine who is in most need of services. Jean Lloyd, the national nutritionist from AoA, referred to a Government Accountability Office (GAO) report (GAO, 2011) that indicated the Aging Network was not reaching the majority of people experiencing food insecurity or social isolation. However, given AoA funding and the necessary prioritization of older adults in need, Lloyd said that AoA is touching those in greatest need.

THE IMPORTANCE OF NUTRITION CARE IN THE COMMUNITY SETTING: CASE STUDY

Presenter: Elizabeth B. Landon

Elizabeth Landon, workshop planning committee member and Vice President of Community Services for CareLink, which represents the Area Agency on Aging for central Arkansas, presented a case study of one of their clients.

George is a 69-year-old veteran who lives alone. He was referred for Meals On Wheels through a hospital discharge meals program because he was very underweight and unable to gain weight. George was on oxygen continuously due to chronic obstructive pulmonary disease. His initial assessment yielded a nutrition risk score of 11 out of 19, with a score of 6 considered high nutrition risk. George was placed in the Meals On Wheels program, which included a daily telephone reassurance call to check on him and monthly nutrition education. However, as with many of CareLink's clients, George needed more than just a meal. A dietitian helped George with a diet plan to gain weight and recommended that he use a nutrition supplement. She also referred him to other services and resources that would benefit him. George said he was unable to afford the nutrition supplement or food and medications, so he was assigned a care coordinator with the meal program to help him.

He received $967 a month from Social Security Income—an income only $60 more a month than the poverty level. Although George had a Medicare prescription drug plan and qualified for a low-income subsidy, each of his 13 prescriptions required a copay from him which he could not afford; therefore, he did not take all of his medications. Furthermore, he had a $25,000 outstanding medical bill.

The care coordinator applied for and received Medicaid Spend-Down[1] for George, which paid the $25,000 outstanding medical bill. She also obtained food stamps for him. Additionally, she applied for the Medicare Savings Program Specified Low Income Medicare Beneficiary, eliminating the copays on all 13 prescriptions and reimbursing the Medicare Part B insurance premiums that had been deducted from George's Social Security Income check. These benefits allowed George to have $110 to spend monthly on the nutrition supplement and other necessities.

George gained 10 pounds in 6 months and improved his nutrition risk score to 5. Even though he is still at risk, he is able to live more comfortably in his own home and, because of these interventions, has not been hospitalized for 16 months. This case illustrates the key role of nutrition intervention in at-risk older people. Landon said that every day this story is repeated across America. One in 11 older people is at risk for hunger every day due to reasons such as chronic poor health, inability to shop or cook, limited income, isolation, or depression (Ziliak and Gundersen, 2011). Unfortunately, many people in similar situations are not benefiting from such services.

REFERENCES

AoA (Administration on Aging). 2010. *A Profile of Older Americans: 2010*. Washington, DC: HHS/AoA. http://www.aoa.gov/aoaroot/aging_statistics/Profile/2010/docs/2010profile. pdf (accessed December 12, 2011).

AoA. 2011a. *About AoA*. http://www.aoa.gov/AoARoot/About/index.aspx (accessed December 13, 2011).

AoA. 2011b. *U.S. OAA 2009 Participant Survey Results*. http://www.state.ia.us/government/ dea/Documents/Nutrition/HealthyAgingUpdate/HealthyAgingUpdate6.2.pdf (accessed December 13, 2011).

GAO (U.S. Government Accountability Office). 2011. *Testimony Before the U.S. Senate Subcommittee on Primary Health and Aging, Committee on Health, Education, Labor, and Pensions: Nutrition Assistance: Additional Efficiencies Could Improve Services to Older Adults*. Washington, DC: GAO. http://www.gao.gov/new.items/d11782t.pdf (accessed December 13, 2011).

---

[1]The process of spending down one's assets to qualify for Medicaid. To qualify for Medicaid Spend-Down, a large part of one's income must be spent on medical care.

HHS (Department of Health and Human Services). 2012. *Administration on Aging: Justifica-*
tion of Estimates for Appropriations Committee, Fiscal Year 2013. Washington, DC:
HHS. http://www.aoa.gov/aoaroot/about/Budget/DOCS/FY_2013_AoA_CJ_Feb_2012.
pdf (accessed February 14, 2012).

NCHS (National Center for Health Statistics). 2011. *Health, United States, 2010: With Special*
Feature on Death and Dying. Hyattsville, MD: CDC/NCHS. http://www.cdc.gov/nchs/
data/hus/hus10.pdf#022 (accessed December 12, 2011).

United Nations Department of Economic and Social Affairs, Population Division. 2010. *World*
Population Ageing 2009. New York: United Nations Department of Economic and Social
Affairs, Population Division.

U.S. Census Bureau. 2011. *Age and Sex Composition: 2010*. Washington, DC: U.S. Census
Bureau. http://www.census.gov/prod/cen2010/briefs/c2010br-03.pdf (accessed December
12, 2011).

Walker, E. L. 2011. The aging landscape in the community setting. Presented at the Institute
of Medicine Workshop on Nutrition and Healthy Aging in the Community. Washington
DC, October 5–6.

Ziliak, J., and C. Gundersen. 2011. *Food Insecurity Among Older Adults: Policy Brief*.
Washington, DC: AARP. http://drivetoendhunger.org/downloads/AARP_Hunger_Brief.
pdf (accessed November 15, 2011).

2

Nutrition Issues of Concern
in the Community

Presenters during the first session provided background on nutrition issues that characterize the needs of older adults who would benefit from community-based nutrition services, said moderator Connie W. Bales, professor of medicine at the Duke University School of Medicine and associate director for education/evaluation at the Durham Veterans Adminstration's Geriatric Research, Education, and Clinical Center. Attention to the issues of nutrition screening, food insecurity, sarcopenic obesity, and dietary patterns, along with supportive community resources, can contribute to improved functionality, independence, and quality of life for older adults.

NUTRITION SCREENING AT DISCHARGE
AND IN THE COMMUNITY
Presenter: Joseph R. Sharkey

Joseph Sharkey, professor of social and behavioral health at the Texas A&M Health Sciences Center, drew on his research with home-delivered meal participants and providers in North Carolina and Texas to discuss nutrition screening and its role in community-based programs within the Aging Network and potential partners. Screening can be a vital part of reaching the national goal of eliminating nutritional health disparities, preventing and delaying chronic disease and disease-related consequences, and improving postdischarge recovery, daily functioning, and quality of life. He

15

discussed nutrition screening versus assessment, challenges associated with screening, determinants of nutritional risk, and uses for nutrition screens.

Nutrition Screening Versus Assessment

Sharkey began by clarifying the difference between nutrition screening and assessment. Screening is used to identify characteristics associated with dietary or nutrition problems, and to differentiate those at high risk for nutrition problems who should be referred for further assessment or counseling. Assessment is a measurement of dietary or nutrition-related indicators, such as body mass index or nutrient intake, used to identify the presence, nature, and extent of impaired nutritional status. This information is used to develop an intervention for providing nutritional care.

Sharkey presented the pathway from the presence of a health condition, to impairment, functional limitations, disability, and adverse outcomes (Nagi, 1976; Verbrugge and Jette, 1994) and noted the role that nutrition and screening could play throughout that progression in preventing advancement to the next stage. Additional reasons for conducting nutrition screening are listed in Box 2-1.

Who Should Be Screened?

In the past, the only people screened were nutrition program participants and those seeking nutrition services. "Is that enough," asked Sharkey, "or should screening be used more broadly to identify and pre-empt some individuals' needs?" While screening people in the community may iden-

---

BOX 2-1
Reasons for Conducting Nutrition Screening

- Determine potential need/demand for community programs
- Prioritize services
- Define short- and long-term outcomes
- Identify or develop interventions
- Prepare nutrition care plans
- Make referrals
- Build basis for additional funding
- Engage community partners

SOURCE: Sharkey, 2011.

tify more high-risk individuals, doing so is made difficult by the following contextual challenges:

- *Geography.* Screening and follow-up may be conducted differently in rural versus urban areas.
- *Population shifts.* The population of older adults in rural areas is increasing due to older adults choosing those locations to retire and younger adults leaving to find jobs.
- *Culture and context.* Immigration may result in the development of new communities that require screening to be conducted within the context of that population's culture.
- *Language.* Nutrition providers should employ people who speak the languages of the populations being screened and can translate materials into those languages. For example, there are nuances to the Spanish language that should be considered when the population includes people from different Spanish-speaking countries.
- *Literacy.* Both educational and health literacy should be considered, especially in the context of various immigrant populations.

He also discussed community challenges for the use of screening:

- *Spectrum of vulnerability.* Screening can be used to identify those individuals at the frail end of the spectrum as well as to prevent people from moving along the continuum to that point. Screeners should be trained to provide people at all points with the appropriate nutrition information, counseling, or referrals.
- *Rapid hospital discharge.* Hospital discharge plans may not take into account challenges associated with high-risk individuals' home and community environments or provide linkages to community-based services.
- *Limited/reduced funding.* Community programs have limited resources so it may be challenging for individuals to locate programs that provide the services they need, such as access to healthy food and transportation.
- *Engagement of nontraditional partners.* How can nontraditional partners, such as the Special Supplemental Nutrition Program for Women, Infants, and Children and Federally Qualified Health Centers be engaged to assist with screening?

Determinants of Nutritional Risk

As previously mentioned, the main purpose of nutrition screening is to identify those at high risk for nutritional problems. Screening for nutritional risk includes gathering information on topics that may be thought of as only partially related or unrelated to food and nutrition, such as social support and transportation. Table 2-1 identifies what are or should be components of nutrition screening and determinants of nutritional risk.

In closing, Sharkey encouraged people to consider the use of screening as a component of prevention as well as the associated ethics of screening, "How can one determine someone to be at risk for poor nutritional health and do nothing?"

TABLE 2-1 Components of Nutrition Screening

Component	Determinants of Risk
Material resources	• Adequacy of income and competing demands (other household members and financial demands) • Household environment (e.g., adequate refrigeration and storage) • Food security • Money, resources, and access • Frequency and duration • Individual components • Energy security (e.g., heating oil, air conditioning)
Individual resources	• Individual capacity and complexity of tasks • Social support: familial and extrafamilial • Partnership status • Food preparation and consumption tasks (e.g., opening a jar, lifting a glass) • Depressive symptoms • Life stresses • Meal patterns (e.g., eating breakfast)

Health	• Disease burden
	• Medications
	  — Multiple prescribed and over the counter (number and therapeutic categories)
	  — Practices to reduce or restrict cost
	  — Adherence
	• Oral and chemosensory health (e.g., problems with chewing and swallowing)
	• Depressive symptoms
	• Life stresses

Other	• Acculturation • Transportation • Access to affordable, healthy foods • Access to food programs

SOURCE: Sharkey, 2011.

FOOD INSECURITY AMONG OLDER ADULTS

Presenter: James P. Ziliak

James Ziliak, chair of microeconomics at the University of Kentucky, presented data from research that he and Craig Gundersen, from the University of Illinois, conducted on food security and food assistance among older Americans. Their research examined the extent, distribution, and determinants of food insecurity among older adults, including differences by age, poverty status, race, and presence of grandchildren, and the health and nutritional consequences of food insecurity.

Households are assigned to food security categories based on responses to 18 questions in the Core Food Security Module (CFSM) developed by the U.S. Department of Agriculture (USDA) and administered as part of a supplement to the Current Population Survey. The CFSM includes questions related to conditions and behaviors experienced by households having trouble meeting basic food needs, such as, "Did you or other adults in your household ever cut the size of your meals or skip meals because there wasn't enough money for food?" (FNS, 2000). The number of affirmative responses dictates the household's food security category (see Table 2-2).

Trends in Food Insecurity Among Older Adults, 2001–2009

Ziliak presented analyses of nationally representative data from the December 2001–2009 Supplements to the Current Population Survey (CPS)

TABLE 2-2 Categories of Food Security

Category	Description of Household Condition	Number of Affirmative Responses to CFSM
Fully food secure	No reported indications of food access problems or limitations	0
Marginal food insecurity	One or two reported indications—typically of anxiety over food sufficiency or shortage of food in the house	1 or more
Food insecurity	Reports of reduced quality, variety, or desirability of diet	3 or more
Very low food security	Reports of multiple indications of disrupted eating patterns and reduced food intake	8 or more in households with children 5 or more in households without children

NOTE: CFSM, Core Food Security Module.
SOURCE: Ziliak and Gundersen, 2011.

(U.S. Census Bureau, 2011a) to provide an overview of food insecurity rates among adults ages 40 years and older. CPS data represent the full set of questions from the CFSM and are used to establish official estimates of food insecurity in the United States.

Background on Adult Food Insecurity in the United States

Between 2001 and 2007, food insecurity rates for adults over age 50 years remained relatively constant. There were spikes in the rates after 2007, which Ziliak suggested is a result of the recession (see Figure 2-1). However, while the rates remained relatively constant in the early 2000s, the actual number of people affected by food insecurity increased at a greater rate; the numbers of people who are food insecure and very low food secure increased 40 and 52 percent, respectively. This is probably a reflection of the "aging society" and the growing number of people 50 years and older, said Ziliak.

Food insecurity among older adults is associated with age, poverty level, race, presence of grandchildren in the household, and geography. Among adults over age 40 years, food insecurity is inversely related to age; the highest rates are among persons 40–49 years (15.2 percent) and the lowest rates are among those 60 years and older (7.3 percent). Among adults ages 50 years and older whose incomes are below 200 percent of the poverty line,[1] about 40 percent are marginally food insecure, 23 percent are food insecure, and 10 percent are very low food secure. There was a linear long-term increase in these rates between 2001 and 2009 and no spike in rates after 2007. There was, however, a spike in rates among people whose incomes were greater than 200 percent of the poverty line, suggesting that income is not the only factor affecting an individual's food security status. Food insecurity rates among those living below the poverty line are two to three times higher than the rates among those living above it.

In 2009, food insecurity rates were highest among Hispanics and African Americans age 50 years and older (about 18 percent) and lowest among whites (7 percent). The spike in rates after 2007 was seen among Hispanics, whites, and Asian and Pacific Islanders, while the rates among African Americans exhibited linear increases. There remains a large gap in food insecurity rates between racial groups even after accounting for income differences (Ziliak and Gundersen, 2011).

Discussing the results from his research on multigenerational hunger,

---

[1] In 2009, the Poverty Thresholds were $11,161 for one person under 65 years of age, $10,289 for one person 65 years of age and over, $14,787 for two people, including a householder under 65 years of age, and $14,731 for two people, including a householder 65 years of age and over (U.S. Census Bureau, 2010).

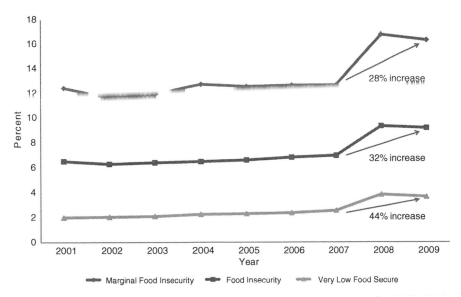

FIGURE 2-1 Food insecurity rates for people ages 50 years and older by level of food insecurity.
SOURCE: Adapted from Ziliak and Gundersen, 2011.

Ziliak showed that the presence of grandchildren in the households of adults 60 years and older is associated with higher rates of food insecurity. In 2009, about 20 percent of adults 60 years and older who had grandchildren in their households were food insecure compared to 7 percent without grandchildren in their households. While these data are more volatile due to the small sample size, rates of food insecurity are on average about three times higher in older adult households with a grandchild present than in those without grandchildren. Ziliak also illustrated the potential destabilizing effect that the presence of a grandchild can have on a food-secure household (see Table 2-3). Regardless of income level, the added presence of a grandchild greatly increases the predicted risk of food insecurity among food secure and insecure households.

"Geographically . . . [food insecurity] is a southern problem," said Ziliak. Rates of food insecurity among adults 50 years and older are highest in the South (7.78 to 12.99 percent) and lowest in the northern Midwest (2.53 to 5.50 percent) (Ziliak and Gundersen, 2011), following the same trend as poverty levels.

After reviewing the data and controlling for other factors, Ziliak and Gundersen found that food insecurity is more likely to affect older adults who

TABLE 2-3 Destabilizing Effect of a Grandchild on Food-Secure and Food-Insecure Households

	Food-Secure Household		Food-Insecure Household	
	Adult over 80 years old, white, retired, married, with a college degree, living in a metro area		Adult 60–64 years old, African American, retired, divorced/separated, did not finish high school, living in a metro area	
	Predicted risk of food insecurity with and without a grandchild present			
Income	No	Yes	No	Yes
< 50% Poverty line	5.8	36.9	53.8	69.6
50–100% Poverty line	5.2	25.8	51.6	57.9
100–200% Poverty line	2.8	21.0	40.5	51.7
> 200% Poverty line	0.6	5.7	19.9	23.2

SOURCE: Analysis of December 2001–2009 Supplements to the Current Population Survey (CPS) data (U.S. Census Bureau, 2011a).

- are living at or below the poverty level,
- do not have a high school degree,
- are African American or Hispanic,
- are divorced or separated,
- have a grandchild living in the household, and
- are younger.

Health Consequences of Food Insecurity

Ziliak and Gundersen reviewed nutrient intake data from the National Health and Nutrition Examination Survey (NHANES) to identify nutrients of concern among adults over 40 years of age. The differences in nutrient intake between food-secure and food-insecure adults in different age groups varies. There are no statistically significant differences in nutrient intake between 40–49-year-old food-secure and food-insecure individuals. Statistically significant differences in nutrient intake in the 50–59-year-old age group were identified for vitamin A, thiamin, vitamin B_6, calcium, phosphorus, magnesium, and iron. However, the differences are not large in magnitude and were no longer present when the sample was restricted to adults below 200 percent of the poverty line. Food-insecure adults over age 60 years have substantially lower intakes of food and all nutrients as compared to food-secure adults in the same age group.

Food-insecure adults ages 50–59 years are more likely than food-secure adults to have limitations in their activities of daily living (ADLs); to be depressed; or to have diabetes; and are less likely to describe their health status as good, very good, or excellent. The gap in health outcomes between food-secure and food-insecure individuals in this age group narrows when the sample is restricted to individuals whose income is below 200 percent of the poverty level. This is due to the increased number of individuals, both food secure and insecure, who have relatively poor health outcomes in this age group and income level.

When controlling for all other factors, Ziliak and Gundersen's multivariate regression models indicate that food-insecure individuals

- ages 50–59 years do not have lower nutrient intakes;
- ages 60 years and older have statistically significant lower nutrient intakes; and
- ages 50 years and older are
    — less likely to be in excellent or very good health,
    — more likely to be depressed, and
    — more likely to have ADL limitations (roughly equivalent to being 14 years older) (Ziliak and Gundersen, 2011).

Concluding Remarks

Ziliak concluded by reiterating the effects that various factors have on food-insecurity rates among older adults in the community and suggesting that they need to be taken into account when developing policy. Rates are highest among 40–49-year-olds, something that should be considered when developing policies for the Supplemental Nutrition Assistance Program (SNAP) since SNAP participation declines with age. Food-insecure individuals over the age of 50 years face serious health consequences; therefore, constructing policies that meet the needs of this population may reduce their risk of negative health outcomes and result in lower health care costs.

SARCOPENIC OBESITY AND AGING

Presenter: Gordon L. Jensen

When the first research on obesity and aging was published over 15 years ago, researchers needed to overcome resistance from geriatricians, said Gordon Jensen, head of the Department of Nutritional Sciences at the Pennsylvania State University. Geriatricians were trained to treat frail older adults in skilled nursing facilities who were underweight, undernourished, and suffering from functional limitations and disability; the idea of obese older adults was new. A great deal has changed in the past 15 years and now many older adults in acute care, transitional care, chronic care, and the community are obese, representing a new population with different health care and nutrition needs.

Obesity and Function Among Older Adults

As with other age groups, obesity is a growing concern among older adults. Data from NHANES 1999–2004 show that the prevalence of obesity among men and women ages 40–79 years is over 30 percent, with rates higher than 40 and 50 percent among Mexican American and black women, respectively (Ogden et al., 2007). The rates may be higher among women because, as Jensen noted, "obese [middle-aged] men tend not to live to be obese older men." Particularly concerning is the relationship between obesity and functional limitations. Elevated current or past body mass index (BMI) has been linked with increased self-reported functional limitations, physical performance testing has confirmed a strong relationship between elevated BMI and functional impairment, and elevated BMI has been associated with increased self-reported homebound status (Jensen, 2005). Predictors of reporting homebound status include

- 75 years of age and older,
- BMI of 35 or greater,
- poor appetite,
- income less than $6,000 a year, and
- limitations in activities of daily living and instrumental activities of daily living (Jensen, 2005).

"These days many older persons in need of services are not tiny and frail; they are large and frail," said Jensen.

Whereas body composition studies have found positive associations between total body fat mass and functional limitations, links between muscle mass and functional limitations have been inconsistent. However, with appropriate adjustment for body size, an association may be detected between relative loss of muscle mass and increased functional limitations (Villareal et al., 2004; Zoico et al., 2004). Obesity is a proxy for sedentary living among older adults because it negatively impacts function. Contributing factors are likely to include obesity's associated medical comorbidities such as diabetes mellitus, hypertension, dyslipidemia, metabolic syndrome, heart disease, and osteoarthritis of the knee. Recent findings further implicate inflammation, sarcopenia, and impairment of muscle function and strength as possibly contributing to functional limitations (Jensen, 2005).

Sarcopenic Obesity

Sarcopenia, the loss of muscle mass with aging, can affect both under- and overweight adults. It can be a major concern for obese older adults since they require more muscle mass to move and function. Loss of α-motor neuron input, changes in insulin hormones, and malnutrition may lead to loss of muscle mass. However, inflammation-driven erosion of muscle mass and a vicious cycle of physical inactivity, increased body fat, and disease burden are likely to culminate in sarcopenic obesity (Jensen and Hsiao, 2010; Stenholm et al., 2008, Zamboni et al., 2008).

Weight Loss Among Obese Older Adults

Although a growing body of research supports consideration of weight loss for some obese older adults, the practice remains controversial. Jensen identified the following reasons (Jensen and Hsaio, 2010):

- Involuntary weight loss usually reflects a serious underlying disease or injury associated with adverse outcomes (Huffman, 2002; McMinn et al., 2011).
- Overweight and mild obesity may be associated with reduced mortality risk (Bouillanne et al., 2009; Curtis et al., 2005).
- Some extra weight may provide a metabolic reserve needed to survive illness or injury (Davenport et al., 2009; Flegal et al., 2007).
- There are concerns for potential losses of muscle and bone mineral density during weight reduction (Chao et al., 2000; Miller and Wolf, 2008; Shapses and Riedt, 2006).

However, findings from weight loss studies suggest that weight loss through exercise and dietary interventions can result in improvements in physical performance testing and functional assessments (Villareal et al., 2006a); reductions in coronary heart disease risk factors such as waist circumference, blood pressure, and glucose, triglyceride, C-reactive protein, and interleukin-6 levels (Villareal et al., 2006b); reductions in the diagnosis of metabolic syndrome (Villareal et al., 2006b); and improvements in systemic and adipose tissue inflammatory states, including reduced levels of C-reactive protein, interleukin-6, and other inflammatory cytokines (Dalmas et al., 2011). A study conducted by Villareal and colleagues (2011) found that a combination of diet and exercise resulted in the greatest improvements in physical function (see Figure 2-2) and diet or a combination of diet and exercise resulted in the most weight loss (see Figure 2-3).

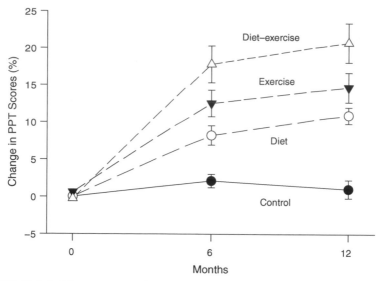

FIGURE 2-2 Mean percent changes in Physical Performance Test (PPT) during intervention.
SOURCE: Villareal et al., 2011. © Massachusetts Medical Society. Reprinted with permission.

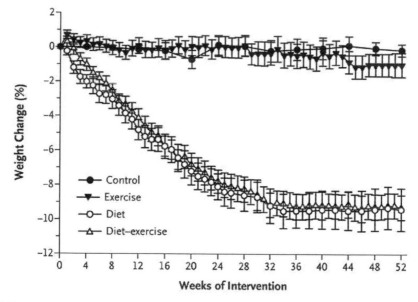

FIGURE 2-3 Mean percent changes in body weight during intervention.
SOURCE: Villareal et al., 2011. © Massachusetts Medical Society. Reprinted with permission.

Weight Status and Nutrient Intake

Jensen presented data from a community-based study of nutrition risk in older persons, further supporting the presence of malnutrition characterized by nutrient deficiencies in obese older adults. Both men and women had inadequate intakes of folate, magnesium, vitamin E, vitamin B_6, zinc, vitamin D, and calcium (Ledikwe et al., 2003). Despite having similar nutrient intakes after adjusting for other factors, only for women were BMI and waist circumference positively associated with intakes of fat and saturated fat and negatively associated with Healthy Eating Index scores and intakes of carbohydrates, fiber, folate, magnesium, iron, and zinc. One explanation for why obese older women were less likely than men to meet nutrient requirements and to have healthy eating patterns may be that older women often live alone whereas men reside with a significant other.

Research Priorities Related to Weight Loss Among Older Adults

In closing, Jensen posed the following questions related to research priorities (Jensen and Hsaio, 2010):

- Which obese older people should be selected for weight reduction?
- What program of prudent diet, behavior modification, and/or exercise is appropriate for which audience?
- What degree of weight loss is appropriate for which audience?
- Are there better approaches to preservation of muscle and bone mineral density during weight reduction?
- For whom is an emphasis on strength and flexibility rather than weight loss the best option?
- Can benefits of weight reduction be maintained in aging subjects?
- Are there anti-inflammatory, resistance training, hormonal, nutritional, or other interventions that may be helpful in preventing or treating sarcopenic obesity?
- Should priority for obese older persons be on diet quality, protein, and micronutrients?

DIETARY INTAKE PATTERNS IN OLDER ADULTS

Presenter: Katherine L. Tucker

Katherine Tucker, professor and chair of the Department of Health Sciences at Northeastern University, explained that individuals' dietary needs change with aging. Older adults may require less energy, experience less efficient absorption and utilization of many nutrients, and have different nutrient requirements due to chronic conditions and medications. These changes result in older adults needing a nutrient-dense diet. Unfortunately, it can be challenging for this population to obtain such a nutrient-dense diet because it involves overcoming barriers such as loss of appetite, changes in taste and smell, oral health decline, mobility constraints, and lower incomes.

Inadequate Intake

Data from the 2003–2004 NHANES were used by the Institute of Medicine Committee to Review Child and Adult Care Food Program Meal Requirements to identify the prevalence of inadequacy of protein and select nutrients among adults 60 years and older (IOM, 2011a) (see Table 2-4). Using NHANES data for adults 70 years and older, Lichtenstein and colleagues (2008) reported calcium, potassium, fiber, and vitamins D, E, and K as shortfall nutrients. In addition to those nutrients, Tucker emphasized the importance of adequate protein intake for prevention of sarcopenia and noted the controversy regarding the current recommendation for protein intake among older adults; should it be the same as the recommendation for younger adults or should it be higher?

TABLE 2-4 Estimated Prevalence of Inadequacy (%) of Protein and Selected Vitamins and Minerals Among Adults ≥ 60 Years Based on Usual Nutrient Intakes from NHANES 2003–2004[a]

Nutrient	Males	Females
Protein	12	20
Vitamin A	54	43
Vitamin C	49	40
Vitamin E	92	98
Thiamin	6.0	12
Riboflavin	2.8	3.7
Niacin	1.8	4.6
Vitamin B_6	19	39
Folate	11	24
Vitamin B_{12}	2.4	9.0
Phosphorus	1.2	4.8
Magnesium	78	73
Iron	1.0	1.5
Zinc	26	21

[a]All nutrients in this table have an Estimated Average Requirement (EAR).
SOURCES: Adapted from IOM, 2011a. Intake data from NHANES 2003–2004. Estimated Average Requirements from Dietary Reference Intake reports (IOM, 1997, 1998, 2000, 2001, 2002/2005).

Tucker highlighted several nutrients of concern in the older adult population.

- *Protein.* The current Estimated Average Requirement for protein for all adults 19 years and older is 0.66 g/kg/day; however, Tucker indicated that a moderately higher protein intake (1.0–1.3 g/kg/day) may be required for older adults to maintain nitrogen balance due to decreased efficiency of protein synthesis and impaired insulin action. Need for increased protein intake is further supported by the Health, Aging, and Body Composition Study, which found that older adults with the highest intake of protein lost less lean body mass than those with lower protein intakes (Houston et al., 2008). However, there is some concern that higher protein intake may increase risk of toxicity or impaired renal function (Paddon-Jones et al., 2008).

- *Vitamin E.* Vitamin E is important because of its role as an antioxidant and in immune function. There is some controversy over whether the current Recommended Daily Allowance, 15 mg of α-tocopherol, is too high, as very few individuals are able to meet this recommendation from diet alone. Vitamin E supplements increase α-tocopherol levels while reducing γ-tocopherol, so supplements may not be the healthiest option for increasing intake. Some literature suggests that other tocopherols (found in nuts, seeds, and plant oils) are also important (Saldeen and Saldeen, 2005); however, there are no current nutrient recommendations for other forms of vitamin E.

- *Vitamin B_{12}.* Although the daily intake of total vitamin B_{12} does not appear to be low for most older adults, dietary intake data may underestimate the number of people who are vitamin B_{12} deficient given that atrophic gastritis and loss of stomach acid prevent some older adults from absorbing it. As a result, the Institute of Medicine (IOM, 2011a) recommended that older adults get their vitamin B_{12} in crystalline form such as from fortified foods or supplements. The Framingham Offspring Study found that nonsupplement users had a higher prevalence of low B_{12} (less than 250 μmol/L) than those who were taking a supplement containing vitamin B_{12} (Tucker et al., 2000). Vitamin B_{12} deficiency can lead to peripheral neuropathy, balance disturbances, cognitive disturbances, physical disability, and increased risk of heart disease from high homocysteine. Tucker stated, "It's critical that more attention be given to this important nutrient as many of these symptoms are nonspecific and not always diagnosed correctly."

- *Vitamin B_6.* Vitamin B_6 is important for numerous metabolic reactions and health outcomes. Inadequacy may lead to high homocysteine and impaired immune function and has been associated with impaired cognitive function and depression. Data from the Massachusetts Hispanic Elders Study showed that 30 percent of Hispanics and 28 percent of non-Hispanic whites had plasma pyridoxal 5′-phosphate (PLP; the active form of vitamin B_6 used as a biomarker for vitamin B_6 status) concentrations less than 30 nmol/L (indicator of inadequate status), and 11 percent of Hispanics and 16 percent of nonwhite Hispanics had concentrations less than 20 nmol/L (clinical cutoff level indicating deficient concentrations). Furthermore, PLP was associated with depressive symptomatology in this population-based study of older adults (Merete et al., 2008).

- *Omega-3 fatty acids.* Among adults 60 years and older, the median intake of α-linolenic acid by women was above the Adequate Intake (AI), whereas the median intake by men was not (IOM, 2011a). Omega-3 fatty acids are associated with protection against heart disease, diabetes, and cognitive decline. Low intake may be partially due to the limited sources in the diet (e.g., fatty fish, flax seeds, and walnuts).

- *Dietary fiber.* Fiber is important for intestinal health and protection against heart disease and metabolic syndrome; however, the median intakes of neither men nor women 60 years and older meet the AI (IOM, 2011a).

- *Vitamin D.* Tucker reported that older adults' poor vitamin D intake and status may be due to low intakes of fortified dairy foods and fatty fish, low sun exposure, reduced dermal synthesis of vitamin D_3 (IOM, 2011b), and decreased capacity of kidneys to convert 25OHD into 1,25-OH_2-D. A study of homebound older adults found that about 65 percent had suboptimal concentrations of 25OHD in their blood (less than 50 nmol/L) and 48 percent had intakes below 400 International Units (Buell et al., 2009). In addition to its importance to bone status, vitamin D deficiency has been associated with neurological conditions, diabetes, and other metabolic conditions. Increasingly, more nutritionists are recommending that older adults take a vitamin D supplement.

Excessive Intakes

Excessive intake of some nutrients is also a concern among older adults as it is for the general population.

- *Sodium.* The Tolerable Upper Intake Level for sodium is 2.3 g/day; however, the 2010 Dietary Guidelines Advisory Committee (DGAC) recommended it should be lowered to 1.5 g/day (HHS and USDA, 2010) to reduce the risk of hypertension and heart disease. Men and women over the age of 70 years are exceeding both recommendations; the usual daily mean intake for men and women is 3.0 and 2.4 g, respectively (IOM, 2010; NHANES 2003 2006).

• *Saturated fat.* The DGAC's 2010 interim recommendation for saturated fat intake is less than 10 percent of energy intake, with the goal of reducing that recommendation to 7 percent (HHS and USDA, 2010). However, most adults have intakes greater than 10 percent of their energy intake (NHANES 2001–2004, 2005–2006).

• *Folic acid.* Whereas some adults do not meet the recommended intake levels of folic acid (400 μg), research shows that others are at risk of exceeding the upper level of 1,000 μg per day due to intake of fortified flour and breakfast cereals, and supplement use. More research is needed but high folic acid may contribute to the progression of neurological diseases associated with vitamin B_{12} deficiency (IOM, 1998) and lead to increased risk of some cancers (Cole et al., 2007; Mason et al., 2007; Stolzenberg-Solomon et al., 2006).

Food Intakes

In order to determine why older adults' nutrient intakes are inadequate, one must review their food intake patterns. The 2011 IOM report *Child and Adult Care Food Programs: Aligning Dietary Guidance for All* presented the mean daily food group intakes by adults ages 60 years and older as compared to the 2,000-calorie MyPyramid food group pattern. It showed that older adults are not meeting any of the MyPyramid food group recommendations and are exceeding the recommendations for daily intake of solid fats and added sugar (see Table 2-5).

Baltimore Longitudinal Study of Aging

The Baltimore Longitudinal Study of Aging collected dietary intake data from 7-day diet records of adults ages 30–80 years old. Five dietary patterns were derived from the data and labeled as follows: "white bread," "healthy," "meat and potatoes," "sweets," and "alcohol." The patterns were based on the foods that contributed the greatest amount of energy to the group; for example, individuals consuming a healthy diet ate more fruit, reduced-fat dairy, and high-fiber cereal. On average, those in the meat and potatoes group had the most gains in BMI over time, those in the white bread group had the largest gains in waist circumference, and those in the healthy group had the smallest gains in both (Newby et al., 2003).

TABLE 2-5 2,000-Calorie MyPyramid Food Group Pattern and Mean
Daily Amounts Consumed by Adults ≥ 60 Years of Age

Food Group or Component	≥ 19 Years 2,000-kcal Pattern[a]	≥ 60 Years Mean Intake[b]
Total fruit (cup eq)	2.0	1.1
Total vegetables (cup eq)	2.5	1.7
Whole grains (oz eq)	3.0	0.86
Total milk group (8 fl oz eq)	3.0	1.3
SoFAS (kcal)	267	570

NOTES: eq, equivalent; fl, fluid; kcal, calories; oz, ounce; SoFAS, solid fats and and sugar.
   [a]Britten et al., 2006.
   [b]NHANES 2003–2004.
SOURCES: Adapted from IOM, 2011a.

Jackson Heart Study

Using similar methods as the Baltimore Longitudinal Study, this study
of African Americans in the southern United States identified different
patterns than those listed above. The most common pattern was the "fast
food pattern"—characterized by fast food, salty snacks, soft drinks, and
meat—which was high in energy, fat, *trans* fat, and saturated fat. The second most common pattern was the "Southern pattern," which consisted
of more cornbread and was high in fat and lower in dietary fiber. The
"prudent pattern" was the least common, reported by only 17 percent of
participants, the majority of which were women (Talegawkar et al., 2008).

Recommendations for Older Adults

Tucker concluded her presentation by recommending some dietary
changes based on the available data. Older adults should be encouraged
to eat

- more fruits and vegetables, especially orange and dark green vegetables, to increase intakes of vitamin C, carotenoids, folate, vitamin
  B_6, magnesium, potassium, and dietary fiber;
- more low-fat dairy to improve intakes of magnesium, calcium,
  potassium, and vitamins B_{12} and D;
- more whole grains, including more fortified breakfast cereals, to
  increase intakes of vitamin B_6, crystalline vitamin B_{12}, magnesium,
  and dietary fiber;
- fewer foods high in sugar, solid fats, sodium; and
- fewer refined grains.

ECONOMIC AND RESOURCE ISSUES SURROUNDING NUTRITION SERVICES FOR OLDER PERSONS IN THE COMMUNITY SETTING

Presenter: Kathryn Larin

Kathryn Larin presented information from two congressionally requested reports developed by the Government Accountability Office (GAO) that focus on nutrition assistance available to older adults. The first report reviewed all of the federally funded nutrition programs in the United States and highlighted the effectiveness of the programs (GAO, 2011a), and the second focused on the Older Americans Act (OAA) Nutrition Program (GAO, 2011b).

Nutrition Assistance Programs Available to Older Adults

GAO's review of the 18 nutrition assistance programs identified four programs that target older adults and three more that are available to the general population but can be accessed by older adults.[2] These programs are listed in Box 2-2.

These programs range in size, reach, amount of federal spending, and types of services provided. Table 2-6 lists the approximate participation in and federal spending on these programs.

Research on the Effectiveness of the Nutrition Assistance Programs

As a part of the report, GAO reviewed the programs' purposes, goals, and the extent to which the goals were being met. While research on these programs is limited, GAO did identify some information on the effectiveness of SNAP and the OAA Nutrition Program.

The goals of the OAA Nutrition Program are to (1) reduce hunger and food insecurity, (2) promote socialization of older individuals, and (3) promote the health and well-being of older individuals through access to nutrition and other disease prevention and health promotion services (AoA, 2011). Studies found that participation in the OAA Nutrition Program resulted in reduced likelihood of food insecurity (Edwards et al., 1993), higher levels of socialization and nutrient intake (Millen et el., 2002), and lower nutrient intakes on days when their meals were not delivered (Sharkey, 2003). Larin said these results are only suggestive because some of

---

[2]Some older adults may be eligible for services through the Community Food Projects Competitive Grant Program; the Food Distribution Program on Indian Reservations; Grants to American Indian, Alaska Native, and Native Hawaiian Organizations for Nutrition and Supportive Services; and the Nutrition Assistance of Puerto Rico.

BOX 2-2
Nutrition Assistance Programs Available to Older Adults

Programs Targeted to Older Adults

- Older Americans Act (OAA) Nutrition Program
- Senior Farmers' Market Nutrition Program
- Commodity Supplemental Food Program (CSFP): adults age 60 years and older who meet income eligibility requirements
- Child and Adult Care Food Program (CACFP): chronically impaired disabled adults and adults age 60 years and older in adult day care centers

Programs That Allow Older Adult Participation

- Supplemental Nutrition Assistance Program (SNAP)
- The Emergency Food Assistance Program (TEFAP)
- The Emergency Food and Shelter National Board Program

TABLE 2-6 Primary Nutrition Assistance Programs Available to Older Adults, FY 2008

Program	Federal Spending (in millions of dollars)	Participation (approximate)
SNAP	37,645.4	28.4 million people 12.7 million households[a]
CACFP	2,394.1	108,000 adults and 3.1 million children[b]
OAA Nutrition Program	745.0	More than 2.5 million seniors
TEFAP	230.6	
Emergency Food and Shelter National Board Program	140.1	73 million meals served
CSFP	100.4	440,000 elderly and 31,000 women, infants, and children[a]
Senior Farmers' Market Nutrition Program	20.1	953,000 low-income seniors

NOTES: CACFP, Children and Adult Care Food Program; CSFP, Commodity Supplemental Food Program; FY, fiscal year; OAA, Older Americans Act; SNAP, Supplemental Nutrition Assistance Program; TEFAP, The Emergency Food Assistance Program.

[a]Average per month.
[b]Average per day.
SOURCE: Consolidated Federal Funds Report, FY 2008.

this research was conducted on pilot or demonstration programs that may not reflect the manner in which the program operates at the national level.

Studies on SNAP found that participation increases household food expenditures (ERS, 2004), increases nutrient availability to households (ERS, 2004), and may reduce anemia and other nutritional deficiencies (Lee et al., 2006). However, research on SNAP generally finds impact at the household level and has found little impact of participation on individuals' dietary or nutrient intake, possibly because not all individuals share equally in SNAP benefits. Furthermore, there has been no SNAP research focused on older adult participants.

Despite the minimal research on the effectiveness of the OAA Nutrition Program, that which is available identifies possible ways to strengthen the program. Research suggests that providing home-delivered breakfast in addition to lunch may increase levels of food security and result in increased intake of calories, protein, carbohydrates, fiber, and minerals by participants (Gollub and Weddle, 2004). In addition, participants' caloric and nutrient intakes could also be increased by delivering "enhanced" energy-dense meals (Silver et al., 2008). However, Larin reiterated that research is limited and dated and that further research on both congregate and home-delivered meals is needed to determine effectiveness. Research on pilot programs may also be beneficial to identify model programs.

Overlap, Duplication, and Fragmentation in Nutrition Assistance Programs

In response to a federal mandate (GAO, 2011c), GAO reviewed nutrition assistance programs to identify areas of program overlap, duplication, and fragmentation. Overlap and duplication are evidenced by multiple programs providing similar services to the same population, while fragmentation is the provision of services through multiple agencies at the federal, state, and local levels. GAO found that the OAA Nutrition Program and Commodity Supplemental Food Program (CSFP) both target older adults, CSFP and The Emergency Food Assistance Program provide similar benefits, and older adults may participate in several programs simultaneously. While providers perceive overlap and duplication as beneficial because it provides multiple points of access and increases the chance that those needing services will obtain them, it may also result in increased administrative costs, inefficient use of federal funding, and confusion among participants and providers.

GAO Report on the OAA Elderly Nutrition Program

GAO analysis of the December Current Population Survey Food Security Supplement shows that among low-income older adult households (age

60 years and older with incomes less than 185 percent of the poverty level), 8.6 percent are food insecure; of these, 5.3 percent have low food security, and 3.3 percent have very low food security (GAO, 2011a). Larin suggested that these numbers likely reflect older adults who need nutrition assistance but are not participating in the programs. Table 2-7 shows the percentage of low-income adults that had characteristics associated with need for nutrition services and the percentages who did and did not receive those services. Larin highlighted the approximately 89 percent of food-insecure older adults that received neither home-delivered nor congregate meals.

Larin suggested that older adults may not be participating in the programs because they

- have limited awareness of available services;
- live in areas with limited available services;
- receive informal services through friends, family, or other organizations;
- choose not to obtain government assistance; or
- receive nutrition assistance through other federal programs, such as SNAP.

Increased Demand for OAA Elderly Nutrition Program Services

A GAO survey of local agencies conducted in the summer of 2010 reports that requests for home-delivered and congregate meals have increased 79 and 47 percent, respectively, since the start of the economic downturn in late 2007. Officials suggest that the increased requests for meals reflects the growing number of adults 60 years and older (greater than than 11 million more Americans were 60 years and older in 2010 than in 2000 [U.S. Census Bureau, 2011b]) and the increasing number of older adults staying in their homes rather than moving to assisted living facilities.

Unfortunately, Larin stated, the growing need for meal services, particularly home-delivered meals, surpasses available resources. While the congregate meal program served more clients in fiscal year (FY) 2008 than the home-delivered meal program, data reflect increasing requests for home-delivered meals. Twenty-two percent of the agencies surveyed by GAO reported being unable to serve all the clients who requested home-delivered meals compared to 5 percent of agencies expressing the same concern about congregate meals. This is in line with data from the Congressional Research Service showing that between 1999 and 2008 the number of congregate meals served decreased by 34 percent while the number of home-delivered meals increased by 44 percent (CRS, 2010). In order to meet this changing need, local programs are shifting funding from congregate meals to home-delivered meals; each year between FY 2000 and FY 2008 the states collec-

TABLE 2-7 Percentage of Low-Income Older Adults[a] with Each Characteristic of Likely Need for Meals Services and Percentages Who Did and Did Not Receive Meals Services

Characteristic of Likely Need	Have Each Characteristic	Received Home-Delivered Meals	Did Not Receive Home-Delivered Meals	Received Congregate Meals	Did Not Receive Congregate Meals	Received Either Type of Meal	Received Neither Type of Meal
Food security							
Food secure	81.4	3.3	96.7	5.7	94.3	8.3	91.7
Food insecure	18.6	7.4	92.6	4.9	95.1	11.1	88.9
Numbers of difficulties with daily activities							
None	65.2	2.3	97.7	5.1	94.9	6.9	93.1
One	18.0	3.6	96.4	6.3	93.7	8.8	91.2
Two or more	16.8	11.5	88.5	6.4	93.6	16.7	83.3
Social isolation[b]							
Less isolated	31.8	2.5	97.5	6.1	93.9	7.9	92.1
More isolated	41.4	5.0	95.0	5.0	95.0	9.0	91.0
Missing[c]	26.8	4.5	95.5	5.8	94.2	9.7	90.3

[a]Adults over the age of 60 years whose incomes were below 185 percent of the poverty level.

[b]Likely need for more social interactions was defined as a response of "no" to all Current Population Survey civic engagement supplement questions about the older adult's participation in social activities. However, such survey data cannot capture more qualitative aspects of an individual older adult's likely need.

[c]Approximately 27 percent of the older adults with low incomes in the sample provided information about participation in meals programs, but not about participation in social groups.

SOURCE: GAO, 2011a. Analysis of December 2008 Current Population Survey Food Security Supplement data.

tively transferred $67 million out of the congregate meal program and into other OAA programs, such as home-delivered meals and support services (GAO, 2011b). Despite the growing need for nutrition services, funding decreased for all programs in 2010, resulting in many programs reducing operational and administrative costs and services.

Closing Comments

Over $90 billion a year is currently spent on nutrition assistance programs, including multiple programs providing services to older adults. Research shows that some of these programs are effectively addressing older adults' nutritional and social needs, yet more updated research is needed to provide additional effectiveness data and to identify services to meet older adults' changing needs. Unfortunately, while need for these programs continues to increase, funding will only continue to decrease in the current budgetary environment. Therefore, it is important that further research identifies and reduces overlap, duplication, and fragmentation of services so funds can be used efficiently.

DISCUSSION

Moderator: Connie W. Bales

During the discussion, points raised by participants included the importance of breakfast, vitamin B_{12} intake, food insecurity, the role of SNAP, and socioeconomic status and food patterns.

The Importance of Breakfast

In response to a request from Robert Miller, Sharkey expanded on the importance of breakfast by stating that consumption of a regular breakfast "jump-started the metabolism for the day" and resulted in increased intake of calcium, vitamin D, magnesium, and phosphorus. Older adults who received breakfast and lunch delivered to their homes consumed more calories, protein, carbohydrates, fiber, and minerals than those who only received lunch, said Larin. Nancy Wellman said that breakfast is one of the easier meals for older adults to assemble; therefore, they should be encouraged to eat that meal at some point during the day.

Crystalline Vitamin B$_{12}$ Intake

Melanie Polk raised the issue of vitamin B$_{12}$ absorption among individuals who are on chronic use of proton pump inhibitors for gastroesophageal reflux disease. Tucker noted that one of the reasons so many older adults are diagnosed as vitamin B$_{12}$ deficient is due to the use of these proton pump inhibitors. However, studies show that some crystalline vitamin B$_{12}$ will be absorbed even in those taking proton pump inhibitors if given in large enough doses.

Food Insecurity Among Older Adult Households with Grandchildren Present

Elizabeth Walker asked why the presence of a grandchild in an older adult's household is associated with higher food insecurity. She wondered whether it was related to the grandparents acting as the primary caregivers or simply due to children being given first choice of the available foods before the adults? Ziliak explained that he and Gundersen are currently examining the health consequences associated with multigenerational food insecurity and will have more results in the near future. The results he presented during the workshop are based solely on the presence of a grandchild, and findings suggest that food insecurity is associated with "the additional anxiety of trying to provide for multiple other individuals [on] a very fixed income." After controlling for income, "on average the presence of a grandchild increases that risk [of food insecurity] by about 50 percent, whether the parent is there or not."

Wellman said that the percent of grandparents caring for a grandchild is fairly low, and Ziliak confirmed that it is probably around 3 to 5 percent; however, there are substantial differences between races and the rate is probably closer to 15 percent in African American households. Sharkey suggested further research to determine food distribution in households where grandparents are present but are not the primary caregivers for the children.

Role of SNAP Among Older Adults

In response to a request from Julie Locher for more information on the role of SNAP in addressing food security among older adults, Larin noted that SNAP is underutilized by older adults. They have the lowest participation rates in SNAP, possibly since they are only eligible for the minimum benefit ($14–$16 per month). Ziliak said, although he cannot prove causality, SNAP participants are at a greater risk of food insecurity and more research needs to be done on that relationship.

Socioeconomic Status and Food Patterns

Charlene Compher inquired about the association between socio-economic status and dietary patterns. Tucker confirmed this association; she noted that people with limited resources are more likely to choose high-calorie, highly refined, high-sugar foods because they are generally less expensive. Diets comprising fruits and vegetables, low-fat dairy foods, and lean meats are more expensive, less widely available, and heavier to carry, all of which may prevent low-income older adults from purchasing them.

NUTRITION ISSUES RELATED TO AGING IN THE COMMUNITY: PERSPECTIVES AND DISCUSSION

Moderator: Gordon Jensen

In the final session of the morning, several speakers representing the workshop sponsoring agencies provided perspectives on nutrition issues of concern related to aging in the community. The moderator, Gordon Jensen, encouraged presenters to discuss important nutritional needs for older adults that differ from those of the community, gaps in services for older adults choosing to stay in their homes, and promising actions for addressing the unique needs to this population.

A Perspective from Abbott Nutrition

Robert Miller, Divisional Vice President of Global Research and Development and Scientific Affairs at Abbott Nutrition, asked "how does [the industry] get nutrition to those people that most need it?" He pointed to the lack of data from intervention studies needed to demonstrate nutrition's impact and stressed the importance of more research to track the effects of nutrition education and supplementation.

In 2010, about 15 percent of hospital patients received nutrition supplementation, the same percent as in 2000. Initial reviews of data suggest that people receiving nutritional supplementation have shorter hospital stays and lower rates of readmission, resulting in lower health care costs. Clinical trials should be used to translate research into something that can be implemented by industry, Miller said. For example, Abbott conducted a pilot study to determine the effect of a nutrition screening and education initiative on hospital readmission rates. The 30-day readmission rate of the 1,000 people followed over 6 months was 8.7 percent, compared to about 24 percent for the area average and 26 percent for the national average. "One of the most simple things in a doctor's bag is education and nutrition

. . . and how do we bring everything from payer, industry, manufacturer, academics, [and] government together to tackle this," Miller concluded.

A Perspective from the Administration on Aging

Jean Lloyd, national nutritionist for the Administration on Aging (AoA), expanded on previous presentations' discussion of the OAA Nutrition Programs. "Although we've talked primarily about the fact that meals are our primary service, it's not just a meals program; it is a nutrition program . . . not a malnutrition program." In efforts to meet the program's three goals (see earlier discussion in this chapter), each year about 50 million meals are home delivered (about 170 meals per participant) and 92.5 million congregate meals are served (about 55 meals per participant). Due to limited government funding, the number of meals served each year has declined; federal funds account for only about 28 percent of the expenditure for home-delivered meals and 41 percent for congregate meals.

In addition to providing meals that meet the current dietary guidelines, the OAA Nutrition Program also includes nutrition education and counseling. The OAA, Lloyd said, provides the opportunity for collaboration among various assistance programs in parallel systems, such as Medicaid waiver programs and the Veterans Administration, in order to develop "comprehensive and coordinated service systems" to meet the nutrition needs of older adults. Despite the success of the program in meeting the needs of this complex and vulnerable population, AoA still faces funding and service cuts and limited nutrition expertise in sites across the country. However, AoA is committed to continuing to improve the way it provides services by conducting research to better understand the needs of its service population. Future plans include conducting outcomes research in the field, administration of process improvement surveys, and research of short-term methods for reducing food insecurity. As a long-term goal, AoA will be conducting impact studies that include reviews of Medicare records for data on emergency room visits and hospitalizations among participants and nonparticipants.

A Perspective from Meals On Wheels Association of America and Meals On Wheels Association of America Research Foundation: The Hidden Hungry

"Over the past 21 years, which is as long as I have been with [Meals On Wheels Association of America], I have become something of an authority on what we at Meals On Wheels Association of America call the 'hidden hungry,'" said Enid Borden, president and Chief Executive Officer. She travels across the country, speaks with people who are "living behind

closed doors," gives them meals, and, most important, listens to their sto-
ries. These older adults may live in the community, but they often stand
apart from it and are overlooked. She hoped her presentation would help
the audience get to know the population being served by giving these older
adults a "human face and voice."

Older adults needing nutrition services are often overlooked by the
community in which they live. She described a trip to a town in Arkansas
with a population of 117 that had become a food desert.[3] She met an
86-year-old woman that had lived there all her life in the house where she
was born. This woman was all alone except for the Meals On Wheels volunteer who delivered her meals. Borden said, "She told me that if it weren't
for Meals On Wheels, she would be dead. She was right."

DISCUSSION

Moderator: Gordon Jensen

During the discussion, points raised by participants included information for case managers, research steps, and aging in place.

Information for Case Managers

Heather Keller inquired about information that case managers should
have to help them determine if they are missing people at nutrition risk.
Lloyd responded that many tools used by case managers do not include
a nutrition component, with the exception of obtaining information on
special diets or nutrition needs based on ADLs. She suggested that case
managers find out more about a person's weight history, appetite, income,
oral conditions, and instrumental ADLs (e.g., shopping for and preparing
meals) and correlate them with responses to food insecurity and functionality questions.

Research Gaps

Robert Russell noted that a real research gap is the lack of analysis
of Medicare and Medicaid records to track the effectiveness of interventions on preventing hospital admissions and readmissions. He asked how

---

[3]The *Food, Conservation, and Energy Act of 2008* (also known as the Farm Bill) (HR 6124,
Sec. 7527) defines a food desert as "an area in the United States with limited access to affordable and nutritious food, particularly such an area composed of predominantly lower-income
neighborhoods and communities."

this would be done by AoA considering differences between programs in various regions of the country; would it be a nationwide evaluation or a review of a selection of similar programs? Lloyd responded that it will be a nationwide evaluation that includes process surveys conducted in all state units on aging, about half of the area agencies on aging, and local providers. The statistical method is still being finalized, but the evaluation will include meal cost at the local level to compare the cost of preparing meals different ways in various parts of the country and a comparison of Medicare data from participants and nonparticipants with different racial and ethnic backgrounds in the same community.

Aging in Place

Katherine Tallmadge pointed out that many communities are organizing groups focusing on aging in place, but wondered if there were any regulations ensuring that people in those groups receive appropriate nutritional care, such as having them track their weight and food intake for consultation with a dietitian. Since those organizations are locally funded and organized and receive no federal funds, the community decides on the requirements, said Lloyd.

Lloyd also addressed the larger issue of programs designed to help keep older adults in their homes. Medicaid funds home- and community-based waivers that are used to keep people out of nursing homes. It is a person-centered program and there are no nutrition or food requirements; however, the states have the option of including them. Over half the states offer a meal service under the waiver program and some states include nutritional supplements and other nutrition services.

REFERENCES

AoA (Administration on Aging). 2011. *Home & Community Based Long-Term Care: Nutrition Services (OAA Title IIIC).* http://www.aoa.gov/aoaroot/aoa_programs/hcltc/nutrition_services/index.aspx (accessed November 14, 2011).

Bouillanne, O., C. Dupont-Belmont, P. Hay, B. Hamon-Vilcot, L. Cynober, and C. Aussel. 2009. Fat mass protects hospitalized elderly persons against morbidity and mortality. *American Journal of Clinical Nutrition* 90(3):505–510.

Britten, P., K. Marcoe, S. Yamini, and C. Davis. 2006. Development of food intake patterns for the MyPyramid Food Guidance System. *Journal of Nutrition Education and Behavior* 38(6 Suppl):S78–S92.

Buell, J. S., T. M. Scott, B. Dawson-Hughes, G. E. Dallal, I. H. Rosenberg, M. F. Folstein, and K. L. Tucker. 2009. Vitamin D is associated with cognitive function in elders receiving home health services. *Journal of Gerontology—Series A Biological Sciences and Medical Sciences* 64(8):888–895.

Chao, D., M. A. Espeland, D. Farmer, T. C. Register, L. Lenchik, W. B. Applegate, and W. H. Ettinger Jr. 2000. Effect of voluntary weight loss on bone mineral density in older overweight women. *Journal of the American Geriatrics Society* 48(7):753–759.

Cole, B. F., J. A. Baron, R. S. Sandler, R. W. Haile, D. J. Ahnen, R. S. Bresalier, G. McKeown-Eyssen, R. W. Summers, R. I. Rothstein, C. A. Burke, D. C. Snover, T. R. Church, J. I. Allen, D. J. Robertson, G. J. Beck, J. H. Bond, T. Byers, J. S. Mandel, L. A. Mott, L. H. Pearson, E. L. Barry, J. R. Rees, N. Marcon, F. Saibil, P. M. Ueland, and E. R. Greenberg. 2007. Folic acid for the prevention of colorectal adenomas: A randomized clinical trial. *Journal of the American Medical Association* 297(21):2351–2359.

CRS (Congressional Research Service). 2010. *Older Americans Act: Title III Nutrition Services Program.* http://aging.senate.gov/crs/nutrition1.pdf (accessed October 10, 2011).

Curtis, J. P., J. G. Selter, Y. Wang, S. S. Rathore, I. S. Jovin, F. Jadbabaie, M. Kosiborod, E. L. Portnay, S. I. Sokol, F. Bader, and H. M. Krumholz. 2005. The obesity paradox: Body mass index and outcomes in patients with heart failure. *Archives of Internal Medicine* 165(1):55–61.

Dalmas, E., C. Rouault, M. Abdennour, C. Rovere, S. Rizkalla, A. Bar-Hen, J. L. Nahon, J. L. Bouillot, M. Guerre-Millo, K. Clément, and C. Poitou. 2011. Variations in circulating inflammatory factors are related to changes in calorie and carbohydrate intakes early in the course of surgery-induced weight reduction. *American Journal of Clinical Nutrition* 94(2):450–458.

Davenport, D. L., E. S. Xenos, P. Hosokawa, J. Radford, W. G. Henderson, and E. D. Endean. 2009. The influence of body mass index obesity status on vascular surgery 30-day morbidity and mortality. *Journal of Vascular Surgery* 49(1):140–147, 147.e1.

Edwards, D. L., E. A. Frongillo Jr., B. A. Rauschenbach, and D. A. Roe. 1993. Home-delivered meals benefit the diabetic elderly. *Journal of the American Dietetic Association* 93(5):585–587.

ERS (Economic Research Service). 2004. *Effects of Food Assistance and Nutrition Programs on Nutrition and Health: Volume 3, Literature Review.* Washington, DC: ERS, USDA. http://www.ers.usda.gov/publications/fanrr19-3/fanrr19-3.pdf (accessed November 15, 2011).

Flegal, K. M., B. I. Graubard, D. F. Williamson, and M. H. Gail. 2007. Cause-specific excess deaths associated with underweight, overweight, and obesity. *Journal of the American Medical Association* 298(17):2028–2037.

FNS (Food and Nutrition Service). 2000. *Guide to Measuring Household Food Security.* Alexandria, VA: FNS, USDA. http://www.fns.usda.gov/fsec/files/fsguide.pdf (accessed November 15, 2011).

GAO (Government Accountability Office). 2011a. *Nutrition Assistance: Additional Efficiencies Could Improve Services to Older Adults.* Washington, DC: GAO. http://www.gao.gov/new.items/d11782t.pdf (accessed November 15, 2011).

GAO. 2011b. *Older Americans Act: More Should Be Done to Measure the Extent of Unmet Need for Services.* Washington, DC: GAO. http://www.gao.gov/new.items/d11237.pdf (accessed December 15, 2011).

GAO. 2011c. *Opportunities to Reduce Potential Duplication in Government Programs, Save Tax Dollars, and Enhance Revenue.* Washington, DC: GAO. http://www.gao.gov/new.items/d11318sp.pdf (accessed November 29, 2011).

Gollub, E. A., and D. O. Weddle. 2004. Improvements in nutritional intake and quality of life among frail homebound older adults receiving home-delivered breakfast and lunch. *Journal of the American Dietetic Association* 104(8):1227–1235.

HHS and USDA (U.S. Department of Health and Human Services and U.S. Department of Agriculture). 2010. *Report of the Dietary Guidelines Advisory Committee on the Dietary Guidelines for Americans, 2010.* http://www.cnpp.usda.gov/Publications/DietaryGuidelines/2010/DGAC/Report/2010DGACReport-camera-ready-Jan11-11.pdf (accessed November 15, 2011).

Houston, D. K., B. J. Nicklas, J. Ding, T. B. Harris, F. A. Tylavsky, A. B. Newman, J. S. Lee, N. R. Sahyoun, M. Visser, and S. B. Kritchevsky. 2008. Dietary protein intake is associated with lean mass change in older, community-dwelling adults: The Health, Aging, and Body Composition (Health ABC) study. *American Journal of Clinical Nutrition* 87(1):150–155.

Huffman, G. B. 2002. Evaluating and treating unintentional weight loss in the elderly. *American Family Physician* 65(4):640–650.

IOM (Institute of Medicine). 1997. *Dietary Reference Intakes for Calcium, Phosphorus, Magnesium, Vitamin D, and Fluoride.* Washington, DC: National Academy Press.

IOM. 1998. *Dietary Reference Intakes for Thiamin, Riboflavin, Niacin, Vitamin B$_6$, Folate, Vitamin B$_{12}$, Pantothenic Acid, Biotin, and Choline.* Washington, DC: National Academy Press.

IOM. 2000. *Dietary Reference Intakes for Vitamin C, Vitamin E, Selenium, and Carotenoids.* Washington, DC: National Academy Press.

IOM. 2001. *Dietary Reference Intakes for Vitamin A, Vitamin K, Arsenic, Boron, Chromium, Copper, Iodine, Iron, Manganese, Molybdenum, Nickel, Silicon, Vanadium, and Zinc.* Washington, DC: National Academy Press.

IOM. 2002/2005. *Dietary Reference Intakes for Energy, Carbohydrate, Fiber, Fat, Fatty Acids, Cholesterol, Protein, and Amino Acids.* Washington, DC: The National Academies Press.

IOM. 2010. *Strategies to Reduce Sodium Intake in the United States.* Washington, DC: The National Academies Press.

IOM. 2011a. *Child and Adult Care Food Program: Aligning Dietary Guidance for All.* Washington, DC: The National Academies Press.

IOM. 2011b. *Dietary Reference Intakes for Calcium and Vitamin D.* Washington, DC: The National Academies Press.

Jensen, G. L. 2005. Obesity and functional decline: Epidemiology and geriatric consequences. *Clinics in Geriatric Medicine* 21(4):677–687.

Jensen, G. L., and P. Y. Hsiao. 2010. Obesity in older adults: Relationship to functional limitation. *Current Opinion in Clinical Nutrition and Metabolic Care* 13(1):46–51.

Ledikwe, J. H., H. Smiciklas-Wright, D. C. Mitchell, G. L. Jensen, J. M. Friedmann, and C. D. Still. 2003. Nutritional risk assessment and obesity in rural older adults: A sex difference. *American Journal of Clinical Nutrition* 77(3):551–558.

Lee, B. J., L. Mackey-Bilaver, and M. Chin. 2006. *Effects of WIC and Food Stamp Program Participation on Child Outcomes.* In *Contractor and Cooperator Report*, 27. Washington, DC: ERS, USDA. http://ddr.nal.usda.gov/bitstream/10113/33688/1/CAT31012177.pdf (accessed November 15, 2011).

Lichtenstein, A. H., H. Rasmussen, W. W. Yu, S. R. Epstein, and R. M. Russell. 2008. Modified MyPyramid for older adults. *Journal of Nutrition* 138(1):5–11.

Mason, J. B., A. Dickstein, P. F. Jacques, P. Haggarty, J. Selhub, G. Dallal, and I. H. Rosenberg. 2007. A temporal association between folic acid fortification and an increase in colorectal cancer rates may be illuminating important biological principles: A hypothesis. *Cancer Epidemiology Biomarkers and Prevention* 16(7):1325–1329.

McMinn, J., C. Steel, and A. Bowman. 2011. Investigation and management of unintentional weight loss in older adults. *British Medical Journal* 342(7800):754–759.

Merete, C., L. M. Falcon, and K. L. Tucker. 2008. Vitamin B6 is associated with depressive symptomatology in Massachusetts elders. *Journal of the American College of Nutrition* 27(3):421–427.

Millen, B. E., J. C. Ohls, M. Ponza, and A. C. McCool. 2002. The Elderly Nutrition Program: An effective national framework for preventive nutrition interventions. *Journal of the American Dietetic Association* 102(2):234–240.

Miller, S. L., and R. R. Wolfe. 2008. The danger of weight loss in the elderly. *Journal of Nutrition, Health and Aging* 12(7):487–491.

Nagi, S. Z. 1976. An epidemiology of disability among adults in the United States. *Milbank Memorial Fund Quarterly, Health and Society* 54(4):439–467.

Newby, P. K., D. Muller, J. Hallfrisch, N. Qiao, R. Andres, and K. L. Tucker. 2003. Dietary patterns and changes in body mass index and waist circumference in adults. *American Journal of Clinical Nutrition* 77(6):1417–1425.

Ogden, C. L., S. Z. Yanovski, M. D. Carroll, and K. M. Flegal. 2007. The epidemiology of obesity. *Gastroenterology* 132(6):2087–2102.

Paddon-Jones, D., K. R. Short, W. W. Campbell, E. Volpi, and R. R. Wolfe. 2008. Role of dietary protein in the sarcopenia of aging. *American Journal of Clinical Nutrition* 87(5):1562S–1566S.

Saldeen, K., and T. Saldeen. 2005. Importance of tocopherols beyond α-tocopherol: Evidence from animal and human studies. *Nutrition Research* 25(10):877–889.

Shapses, S. A., and C. S. Riedt. 2006. Bone, body weight, and weight reduction: What are the concerns? *Journal of Nutrition* 136(6):1453–1456.

Sharkey, J. R. 2003. Risk and presence of food insufficiency are associated with low nutrient intakes and multimorbidity among homebound older women who receive home-delivered meals. *Journal of Nutrition* 133(11):3485–3491.

Sharkey, J. 2011. Nutrition screening at discharge and in the community. Presented at the Institute of Medicine Workshop on Nutrition and Healthy Aging in the Community. Washington DC, October 5–6.

Silver, H. J., M. S. Dietrich, and V. H. Castellanos. 2008. Increased energy density of the home-delivered lunch meal improves 24-hour nutrient intakes in older adults. *Journal of the American Dietetic Association* 108(12):2084–2089.

Stenholm, S., T. B. Harris, T. Rantanen, M. Visser, S. B. Kritchevsky, and L. Ferrucci. 2008. Sarcopenic obesity: Definition, cause and consequences. *Current Opinion in Clinical Nutrition and Metabolic Care* 11(6):693–700.

Stolzenberg-Solomon, R. Z., S. C. Chang, M. F. Leitzmann, K. A. Johnson, C. Johnson, S. S. Buys, R. N. Hoover, and R. G. Ziegler. 2006. Folate intake, alcohol use, and postmenopausal breast cancer risk in the Prostate, Lung, Colorectal, and Ovarian Cancer Screening Trial. *American Journal of Clinical Nutrition* 83(4):895–904.

Talegawkar, S. A., E. J. Johnson, T. C. Carithers, H. A. Taylor Jr., M. L. Bogle, and K. L. Tucker. 2008. Serum carotenoid and tocopherol concentrations vary by dietary pattern among African Americans. *Journal of the American Dietetic Association* 108(12):2013–2020.

Tucker, K. L., S. Rich, I. Rosenberg, P. Jacques, G. Dallal, P. W. F. Wilson, and J. Selhub. 2000. Plasma vitamin B-12 concentrations relate to intake source in the Framingham Offspring Study. *American Journal of Clinical Nutrition* 71(2):514–522.

U.S. Census Bureau. 2010. *Poverty Thresholds 2009.* http://www.census.gov/hhes/www/poverty/data/threshld/thresh09.html (accessed January 11, 2012).

U.S. Census Bureau. 2011a. *Current Population Survey.* http://www.census.gov/cps/ (accessed November 29, 2011).

U.S. Census Bureau. 2011b. *Age and Sex Composition: 2010.* Washington, DC: U.S. Census Bureau. http://www.census.gov/prod/cen2010/briefs/c2010br-03.pdf (accessed November 15, 2011).

Verbrugge, L. M., and A. M. Jette. 1994. The disablement process. *Social Science and Medicine* 38(1):1–14.

Villareal, D. T., M. Banks, C. Siener, D. R. Sinacore, and S. Klein. 2004. Physical frailty and body composition in obese elderly men and women. *Obesity Research* 12(6):913–920.

Villareal, D. T., M. Banks, D. R. Sinacore, C. Siener, and S. Klein. 2006a. Effect of weight loss and exercise on frailty in obese older adults. *Archives of Internal Medicine* 166(8):860–866.

Villareal, D. T., B. V. Miller III, M. Banks, L. Fontana, D. R. Sinacore, and S. Klein. 2006b. Effect of lifestyle intervention on metabolic coronary heart disease risk factors in obese older adults. *American Journal of Clinical Nutrition* 84(6):1317–1323.

Villareal, D. T., S. Chode, N. Parimi, D. R. Sinacore, T. Hilton, R. Armamento-Villareal, N. Napoli, C. Qualls, and K. Shah. 2011. Weight loss, exercise, or both and physical function in obese older adults. *New England Journal of Medicine* 364(13):1218–1229.

Zamboni, M., G. Mazzali, F. Fantin, A. Rossi, and V. Di Francesco. 2008. Sarcopenic obesity: A new category of obesity in the elderly. *Nutrition, Metabolism and Cardiovascular Diseases* 18(5):388–395.

Ziliak, J., and C. Gundersen. 2011. *Food Insecurity Among Older Adults: Policy Brief.* Washington, DC: AARP. http://drivetoendhunger.org/downloads/AARP_Hunger_Brief.pdf (accessed November 15, 2011).

Zoico, E., V. Di Francesco, J. M. Guralnik, G. Mazzali, A. Bortolani, S. Guariento, G. Sergi, O. Bosello, and M. Zamboni. 2004. Physical disability and muscular strength in relation to obesity and different body composition indexes in a sample of healthy elderly women. *International Journal of Obesity* 28(2):234–241.

3

Transitional Care and Beyond

During the second session of the workshop, speakers discussed topics related to providing care for people before, during, and after hospital discharge. They explored the current and potential roles of registered dietitians in hospitals, a multidisciplinary approach to discharge, and home- and community-based services. Hospitalization is common among older adults and they are being discharged sicker than in the past said Nadine Sahyoun, associate professor of nutrition epidemiology at the University of Maryland in College Park, who moderated the session. Transitional care models "follow patients across settings, improve coordination among health care providers, and also help individuals better understand their posthospital care," she said. Nutrition services are an important element of transitional care and recovery to ensure that older adults in their homes are well nourished.

ROLE OF NUTRITION IN HOSPITAL DISCHARGE PLANNING: CURRENT AND POTENTIAL CONTRIBUTION OF THE DIETITIAN

Presenter: Charlene Compher

Charlene Compher, associate professor of nutrition science at the University of Pennsylvania School of Nursing, drew on her experiences in a hospital setting at the Hospital of the University of Pennsylvania (HUP) as context for her presentation. HUP is rated among the top 10 hospitals in the United States, providing trauma, cancer, transplant, cardiac, and geriatric care, yet only had 20 registered dietitians (RDs) to provide nutritional care to the almost 800 patients per day and 42,500 admissions in fiscal year 2011. HUP has a 2014 goal of eliminating preventable deaths and 30-day readmissions, and achieving both requires all hospital employees, including RDs, to focus on the same goals.

The Role of RDs in Hospital Readmissions

In order to achieve its 2014 goal of eliminating 30-day readmissions, HUP will address the factors that predict hospital readmissions, such as those identified in Box 3-1.

There is a growing body of research demonstrating that dietitians can help prevent hospital readmission by providing nutrition counseling that changes patients' behaviors and improves clinical outcomes. Studies have shown that RD counseling can result in weight loss (Raatz et al., 2008), improved weight management and lipid profiles (Gaetke et al., 2006; Welty et al., 2007), sustained heart-healthy diet modifications (Cook et al., 2006), and adherence to a low-sodium diet in patients with heart failure (Arcand et al., 2005). Implementation of recommendations for enteral tube feeding in long-term acute care facility patients resulted in shorter lengths of stay, improved albumin levels, and desired weight gain (Braga et al., 2006). Compher highlighted an "intriguing study" conducted by Feldblum and colleagues in Israel among adults age 65 years and older. Feldblum et al. (2011)

BOX 3-1
Factors that Predict Hospital Readmissions

Utilization Factors

- Longer length of stay
- Prior admission(s) in the past year
- Previous emergency department visits

Patient Characteristics

- Comorbidity (diabetes mellitus, hypertension, congestive heart failure, chronic kidney disease, depression)
- Living alone
- Discharged to home
- Medicare/Medicaid

SOURCE: Leas and Umscheid, 2011.

compared outcomes in a control group receiving the standard in-hospital screen or one visit by an RD to those in the intervention group receiving three home visits by an RD after discharge combined with individualized nutrition assessment, enhanced food intake, and nutrition supplements, as needed. The intervention group scored better on nutritional assessment, experienced less frequent hypoalbuminemia, and had lower mortality rates when compared to the control group. However, Compher noted, results do not indicate if the improvements were due to the nutrition care received in the hospital or the RD visits after discharge, so the results are attributed to both.

The Role of RDs in Current Hospital Nutrition Practice

As required by the Joint Commission, nutrition screening at HUP is completed within 24 hours of hospital admission. A nurse usually completes the screening, which includes individual institutional criteria such as unexpected weight gain or loss, gastrointestinal symptoms, obvious emaciation, pressure ulcers, and home feeding by intravenous or tube route. Patients identified as high risk are referred to an RD for a full nutrition assessment. This assessment, which is more complex and may take more than an hour to complete, includes

- diet history,
- weight history,
- medical history,
- medication profile,
- laboratory values,
- current conditions, and
- physical examination for nutrient deficiency or excess.

Once the assessment is completed, a nutrition care plan is developed and the patient's nutrition risk level is set to establish a follow-up schedule.

RDs also conduct nutrition assessments on people referred by physicians, admitted with a high-risk diagnosis or condition (e.g., receiving care in the intensive care unit), and receiving monitored nutrition support therapy. RDs provide instructions for people being discharged with home tube feeding and parenteral nutrition support, take part in discharge planning rounds, and communicate with RDs in outpatient care centers. Compher remarked that, while it would be ideal to provide nutrition assessment to all patients, the process is time consuming, hospitals have inadequate RD staff, hospital stays are too short, and hospitals' limited resources are used on patients for whom nutrition interventions will provide the best outcomes.

Potential Future RD Roles

Compher suggested that, despite limited time and resources, there are at least three opportunities to improve the ways RDs are involved in preventing hospital readmissions:

1. *Ensure that nutrition assessment goals are included in discharge plans.* Through the use of electronic medical records, patients' nutrition assessment goals and information could be transmitted directly to their discharge plans. This may assist discharge planners in making the appropriate referrals. Ideally, RDs would be included on the discharge planning team to review hospital records for nutrition care plans that require home support, identify people whose nutrition status has changed and who require increased care, and communicate with staff at outside facilities that provide postdischarge care.
2. *Increase cases receiving nutrition assessments.* Compher acknowledged that hospitals may not have the staff, funding, or time to increase the number of people screened and assessed. She suggested using dietetic technicians to conduct the screenings and referrals and to focus on those people most likely to be readmitted, including everyone 65 years and older and patients admitted through the emergency room. She also suggested that dietitians screen patients in the emergency department in order to begin nutrition care early or to identify patients in need of nutrition services although not being admitted and make the necessary referrals.
3. *Improve integration of hospital and post hospital nutrition care.* Although achieving this goal requires more trained nutrition professionals in the community, it would be beneficial to have hospital RDs more involved in post hospital care. Compher proposed having RD positions in heart failure programs, all outpatient clinical programs, and community geriatric care programs. She also suggested paying RDs for home visits to conduct nutrition assessments and providing hospitals with financial incentives for avoiding readmissions.

Closing Comments

Compher concluded by noting the importance of moving from the current level of RD availability into a future with enhanced nutrition care for older adults. It may be daunting but it is imperative that the nutrition community "take the challenge" to prevent hospitals from discharging nutritionally compromised people who are more likely to be readmitted.

TRANSITIONAL CARE: A MULTIDISCIPLINARY APPROACH

Presenter: Eric A. Coleman

Eric Coleman, professor of medicine and head of the Division of Health Care Policy and Research at the University of Colorado at Denver, reiterated the importance of a team approach to providing transitional care, stressing that the most important teammate is the one receiving the care. The ultimate goal for transitional care is "to create a match between the individual's care needs and his or her care setting." Achieving that goal can reduce frequent and costly readmission rates; the Medicare 30-day hospital readmission rate is nearly 20 percent (AHRQ, 2007) and hospitals with high readmission rates are financially penalized under the Affordable Care Act.

The Role of Nutrition in Hospital Readmissions and Transitional Care

While nutrition plays a role in improving general health, the role of nutrition in hospital readmission remains unclear, Coleman said. There are studies linking the two but they mostly explore undernutrition, are observational, sometimes rely on clinical assessment or laboratory results, and rarely explore the role of supplementation (Friedmann et al., 1997). He noted that "the role of nutrition is likely entangled with chronic illness, frailty, [and] socioeconomic status." Nutrition should not be used as a bartering tool in a hospital's efforts to provide intervention in a patient's home, cautioned Coleman. For example, in order to avoid financial penalties, hospitals are eager to intervene on high-risk older adults and may use nutrition services as an incentive to persuade them to agree to home visits.

The Role of the Patient in Transitional Care

In order to determine how to improve the quality of transitional care, Coleman suggested talking to people receiving the services. He said they report feeling unprepared and unsure of what to do when they return home. They are confused because they receive conflicting advice from professionals in various health care settings, and they do not know who to contact to reconcile the discrepancies. Finally, they are frustrated because their family caregivers are left to complete tasks that the professionals left undone. Often people receiving transition services interact with their health care providers for only a few hours a week. Therefore, they, or their family members, end up acting as their own caregivers, making decisions without the skills, tools, or confidence to provide effective care. As shown in Ed Wagner's Chronic Care Model (see Figure 3-1), an informed and active

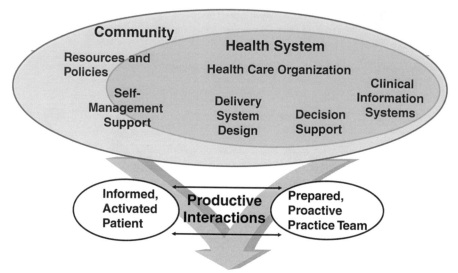

Functional and Clinical Outcomes

FIGURE 3-1 Wagner's Chronic Care Model.
SOURCE: Wagner, 1998. Reprinted, with permission, from the American College of Physicians.

patient is vital to achieving improved functional and clinical outcomes (Wagner, 1998; Wagner et al., 2001).

The Care Transitions Intervention™

The Care Transitions Intervention™ (CTI) is a low-cost, low-intensity intervention designed to build one's skills and confidence and provide the necessary tools to encourage the patient to be an informed and active decision maker during care transitions (Coleman, 2011). The intervention consists of one home visit within 48–72 hours after discharge and three phone calls within 30 days. The patient's "transition coach" models behavior for how to handle common problems, role-plays the next health care visit, elicits the patient's health-related goals to be accomplished in the next 30 days, and creates a comprehensive medication list. Because the patients and caregivers are members of their own interdisciplinary team, they identify their own health care goals and the skills needed to coordinate their care across settings. The four areas that patients identified as those they need the most help with (referred to as the "four pillars") are

1. development of a patient-centered health record,
2. assistance with medication self-management,
3. follow-up with primary care physician and specialists, and
4. knowledge of "red flags" or warning signs and symptoms and how to respond.

The patient-centered health record contains the patient's current medical conditions, warning signs that relate to the patient's condition, a list of medications and allergies, advance directives, and space for the patients to list their questions or concerns to discuss during their next health care visit. The transition coach initially meets with the patient prior to hospital discharge to introduce the program and patient-centered health record, establish rapport, and schedule the home visit. During the home visit, the patient indentifies a 30-day health-related goal; the coach reconciles the patient's medications; and they role-play how to respond to red flags, obtain a timely follow-up appointment, and raise questions for health care providers during subsequent visits. The phone calls are conducted to follow up on active coaching issues, review the four pillars of the intervention, estimate the amount of progress being made, and ensure the patient's needs are being met (Coleman, 2011).

CTI Key Findings and Next Steps

Results from the CTI showed that reductions in hospital readmission rates were significantly lower at 30 days postdischarge (the time period in which the transition was involved). Furthermore, significantly lower rates at 90 and 180 days postdischarge demonstrate the sustained effect of the coaching. The net cost savings for 350 patients over 12 months was $300,000. CTI has been adopted by 500 health care organizations in 38 states and resulted in reduced 30-, 60-, and 80-day readmission rates (Coleman et al., 2004; Crouse Hospital, 2008; Parry et al., 2006; Perloe et al., 2011). Preliminary data from evidence-based care transition grants from the Administration on Aging and the Centers for Medicare & Medicaid Services show that 16 states are employing models to help older adults stay in their homes after discharge from hospitals, rehabilitation centers, or skilled nursing facilities, 11 of which are implementing CTI. In April 2011 up to $500 million was made available by the Secretary of the Department of Health and Human Services under the Affordable Care Act Section 3026 to fund organizations to provide evidence-based transition care services to high-risk Medicare recipients (CMS, 2011).

Closing Remarks

Coleman concluding by summarizing the four factors that promote successful implementation of CTI: (1) model fidelity, (2) selection of an appropriate transition coach, (3) execution of the model, and (4) support to sustain the model. Successful implementation of CTI can reduce readmission rates by helping older adults and their caregivers become informed and active participants in their care transitions.

NUTRITION IN HOME- AND COMMUNITY-BASED SYSTEMS: PERSPECTIVES FROM THE FIELD

Presenter: Bobbie L. Morris

Through her position at the Alabama Department of Senior Services, Bobbie Morris visits older adults in their homes and senior centers and learns about the nutrition services they are receiving. Services provided under the Older Americans Act (OAA) Elderly Nutrition Program aim to promote health, provide nutritious meals that meet current dietary guidelines and older adults' needs, reduce social isolation, and link adults to social rehabilitative services through other home- and community-based long-term care organizations. Her experiences suggest that facilities that promote fun and physical activity in addition to the OAA services of meals, nutrition education, counseling, and screening and assessment may have higher rates of participation.

Services Provided Under Title III C of the OAA Nutrition Program

Under Title III C of the OAA Nutrition Programs, meals can be served through congregate or home-delivered services. Congregate nutrition services provide meals five or more days a week in a group setting, including adult daycare, whereas home-delivered meals are hot, cold, frozen, dried, canned, and supplemental foods that are distributed to adults' homes. In both cases, nutrition education and counseling are provided to the recipients and, in the case of home-delivered meals, their caregivers (AoA, 2011a). The numbers of congregate, home-delivered, and total meals served through the OAA Nutrition Services program over the past 10 years are shown in Table 3-1.

As mentioned in a previous presentation, the number of home-delivered meals has increased over the years while the number of congregate meals has decreased, possibly indicative of the number of frail older adults staying in their homes, Morris said. She suggested that the decline in total meals

TABLE 3-1 Number of Meals Served Through OAA Nutrition Services in the United States

Fiscal Year	Number of Meals Served		
	Home-Delivered Meals	Congregate Meals	Total Meals
2000	143,804,683	116,016,249	259,820,932
2001	143,719,629	112,243,758	255,963,387
2002	141,958,732	108,333,836	250,292,568
2003	142,889,385	105,905,622	248,795,007
2004	143,163,389	105,606,162	248,769,551
2005	140,132,325	100,530,354	240,662,679
2006	140,212,524	98,031,661	238,244,185
2007	140,990,040	94,877,137	235,867,177
2008	146,897,367	94,196,192	241,093,559
2009	149,188,917	92,492,669	241,681,586

NOTE: Data include number of meals served in 50 states, District of Columbia, and U.S. territories.
SOURCE: Data from 2000–2004: AoA, 2009; data from 2005–2009: AoA, 2011b.

served is partially due to increases in fuel and food costs that exceed program funding increases.

Flexible Meals Services

Morris described several flexible meal services funded by a variety of sources. In some cases, meals may be offered at a range of locations and at various times during the day. Voucher programs provide participants with the option to go to a restaurant or grocery store and order a meal or purchase items that meet the required nutrition guidelines. In some areas where there are limited restaurants, hospital vouchers can be used to purchase a meal from a hospital cafeteria. In some areas, meals may also be offered at homeless shelters. Flexible meal packages include options for receiving more than one meal per day, such as a hot meal at lunch and a frozen meal for dinner, or shelf-stable meals for weekends, holidays, and emergencies.

Meals can be provided through local and statewide contracts, at on-site kitchens, and by shipments to participants' homes. For example, a local contract could arrange for a community nursing home or restaurant to prepare and deliver meals to homebound adults or congregate meal facilities. Alabama has a statewide contract with Valley Food Service for preparation of all hot and frozen meals for the state. The benefit of a statewide contract is reduced meal costs; however, it also limits the variety of available foods and results in all state participants receiving the same meal.

Prioritizing Services

Despite the availability of Title III nutrition services and programs like Meals On Wheels, there are still people on waiting lists for meals. The OAA states that "services are targeted to those in greatest social and economic need with particular attention to low-income individuals, minority individuals, those in rural communities, those with limited English proficiency, and those at-risk of institutional care" (AoA, 2011a). In order to determine who is most in need of service, nutrition risk is assessed using tools such as the Nutrition Screening Initiative checklist (Posner et al., 1993) and the Mini Nutritional Assessment® (Nestlé Nutrition Institute, 2011; Vellas et al., 1999). Morris stressed the importance of properly training staff on how to administer the assessment tools to ensure that the questions are asked correctly and the appropriate information obtained. Other ways to determine who on the waiting list receives meals or to provide alternate services include

- decisions made by a Senior Center Advisory Board based on need;
- a first-come, first-served approach;
- sponsored meals provided by organizations such as churches, rotary clubs, and women's clubs; and
- managing delivery routes to redirect meals intended for those who cancelled their meal service to be delivered to other people in the same area.

Closing Remarks

Morris closed by sharing her view that a "no wrong door" philosophy would provide seamless access to services regardless of how or where someone encounters the service system. She suggested that service programs and funding streams be brought together to ensure that older adults receive the information, referrals, and care they need. The long-term goal is for older adults to make informed choices for their long-term care, while reducing and controlling Medicaid spending, decreasing nursing home and institutional care, increasing availability of home- and community-based services, and reducing the number of people on waiting lists for nutrition services.

DISCUSSION

Moderator: Nadine R. Sahyoun

During the discussion, points raised by participants included the role of nutrition in transition services, the role of physicians in the referral process, and patients' perception of needs during and after discharge.

Role of Nutrition in Transition Services

Nancy Wellman questioned why nutrition is not a larger component of transition services. Coleman noted that while nutrition was mentioned during his qualitative research, the focus of the CTI model is patient-identified goals, not those chosen by the health care provider, so nutrition will not be addressed if it is not one of the patient's goals. Rose Ann DiMaria-Ghalili followed up by pointing out that none of the transitional care models published by the Remington Report included a nutrition component. She said this is "quite alarming" and believes nutrition screening should be conducted throughout the transitions. She also suggested that health care professions using various screening tools collaborate to ensure consistency, and nurses would be amenable to using whatever tool is recommended.

Role of Physicians in Referral Process

Jennifer Troyer referred to Compher's statement that two-thirds of referrals to RDs for nutrition assessment were from physicians and wondered if it was the same physicians repeatedly making the referrals. Compher stated that it was a variety of physicians, possibly due to HUP's role as a teaching hospital; residents make referrals following the lead of physicians they respect and continue to refer patients to RDs as they move up the tiered levels of training. Heather Keller asked why more people were not being referred to RDs as a result of the nutrition screening, and why physicians were making the majority of referrals. One-third of HUP's beds are intensive care unit beds; therefore, referrals for those patients are more likely to come from a physician. Coleman noted that hospital stays are shorter and people may be discharged before laboratory results from the nutrition evaluation indicating nutrition problems are received. He said, "if we're going to pursue these evaluations, it's also worth thinking about the workflow, about what happens when the lab comes back abnormal and the person left 24–48 hours ago."

The Patient's Perception of Need During and Postdischarge

James Hester asked about the panelists' experiences understanding patients' perceptions of their needs during discharge and postdischarge, including their receptivity to their nutritional needs. Compher noted that based on her personal experience individuals who are being discharged from the hospital want more than anything to be home and in a situation they understand and can control. Coleman agreed that individuals tend to feel inundated while in the hospital, and suggested letting them get settled in their homes and then addressing some of the issues several weeks later, when they may be more prepared to think about them. Sahyoun added that individuals may have support from their family and friends the first few days after discharge but then there is an adjustment period while they figure out how to handle situations on their own. She suggested "that in the transition of care there is a role to play in making people aware and empowering them [with knowledge] about what [nutrition] resources are available in the community" in addition to other health services.

REFERENCES

AHRQ (Agency for Healthcare Research and Quality). 2007. *Slide Presentation from the AHRQ 2007 Annual Conference: Medicare Hospital 30-Day Readmission Rates and Associated Costs, by Hospital Referral Regions, 2003.* http://ahrq.hhs.gov/about/annualmtg07/0928slides/schoen/Schoen-17.html (accessed December 19, 2011).

AoA (Administration on Aging). 2009. *Aging Integrated Database: State Program Reports (SPR) 2000–2004.* http://classic.agidnet.org/SPR.asp (accessed January 12, 2012).

AoA. 2011a. *Home & Community Based Long-Term Care: Nutrition Services (OAA Title IIIC).* http://www.aoa.gov/aoaroot/aoa_programs/hcltc/nutrition_services/index.aspx (accessed November 14, 2011).

AoA. 2011b. *Aging Integrated Database.* http://www.agidnet.org/ (accessed November 3, 2011).

Arcand, J. A. L., S. Brazel, C. Joliffe, M. Choleva, F. Berkoff, J. P. Allard, and G. E. Newton. 2005. Education by a dietitian in patients with heart failure results in improved adherence with a sodium-restricted diet: A randomized trial. *American Heart Journal* 150(4):716.e1–716.e5.

Braga, J. M., A. Hunt, J. Pope, and E. Molaison. 2006. Implementation of dietitian recommendations for enteral nutrition results in improved outcomes. *Journal of the American Dietetic Association* 106(2):281–284.

CMS (Centers for Medicare & Medicaid Services). 2011. Medicare program; Solicitation for proposals for the Medicare Community-Based Care Transitions Program. *Federal Register* 76(73):21372–21373.

Coleman, E. A. 2011. *The Care Transitions Program®.* http://www.caretransitions.org (accessed December 12, 2011).

Coleman, E., J. Smith, and S. Min. 2004. Post-hospital medication discrepancies: Prevalence, types, and contributing system-level and patient-level factors. *The Gerontologist* 44(1):509–510.

Cook, S. L., R. Nasser, B. L. Comfort, and D. K. Larsen. 2006. Effect of nutrition counselling: On client perceptions and eating behaviour. *Canadian Journal of Dietetic Practice and Research* 67(4):171–177.

Crouse Hospital. 2008. *Crouse Hospital Care Transitions Program.* http://www.caretransitions.org/documents/Crouse_2008.pdf (accessed December 12, 2011).

Feldblum, I., L. German, H. Castel, I. Harman-Boehm, and D. R. Shahar. 2011. Individualized nutritional intervention during and after hospitalization: The nutrition intervention study clinical trial. *Journal of the American Geriatrics Society* 59(1):10–17.

Friedmann, J. M., G. L. Jensen, H. Smiciklas-Wright, and M. A. McCamish. 1997. Predicting early nonelective hospital readmission in nutritionally compromised older adults. *American Journal of Clinical Nutrition* 65(6):1714–1720.

Gaetke, L. M., M. A. Stuart, and H. Truszczynska. 2006. A single nutrition counseling session with a registered dietitian improves short-term clinical outcomes for rural Kentucky patients with chronic diseases. *Journal of the American Dietetic Association* 106(1):109–112.

Leas, B., and C. A. Umscheid. 2011. *Risk Factors for Hospital Readmission.* Philadelphia, PA: Center for Evidence-based Practice.

Nestlé Nutrition Institute. 2011. *MNA® Mini Nutritional Assessment: Overview.* http://www.mna-elderly.com/default.html (accessed November 14, 2011).

Parry, C., H. M. Kramer, and E. A. Coleman. 2006. A qualitative exploration of a patient-centered coaching intervention to improve care transitions in chronically ill older adults. *Home Health Care Services Quarterly* 25(3–4):39–53.

Perloe, M, K. Rask, and M. L. Keberly. 2011. Standardizing the hospital discharge process for patients with heart failure to improve the transition and lower 30 day readmissions. *The Remington Report*, http://www.cfmc.org/integratingcare/files/Remington%20Report%20Nov%202011%20Standardizing%20the%20Hospital%20Discharge.pdf (accessed December 12, 2011).

Posner, B. M., A. M. Jette, K. W. Smith, and D. R. Miller. 1993. Nutrition and health risks in the elderly: The Nutrition Screening Initiative. *American Journal of Public Health* 83(7):972–978.

Raatz, S. K., J. K. Wimmer, C. A. Kwong, and S. D. Sibley. 2008. Intensive diet instruction by registered dietitians improves weight-loss success. *Journal of the American Dietetic Association* 108(1):110–113.

Vellas, B., Y. Guigoz, P. J. Garry, F. Nourhashemi, D. Bennahum, S. Lauque, and J. L. Albarede. 1999. The Mini Nutritional Assessment (MNA) and its use in grading the nutritional state of elderly patients. *Nutrition* 15(2):116–122.

Wagner, E. H. 1998. Chronic disease management: What will it take to improve care for chronic illness? *Effective Clinical Practice* 1(1):2–4.

Wagner, E. H., B. T. Austin, C. Davis, M. Hindmarsh, J. Schaefer, and A. Bonomi. 2001. Improving chronic illness care: Translating evidence into action. *Health Affairs* 20(6):64–78.

Welty, F. K., M. M. Nasca, N. S. Lew, S. Gregoire, and Y. Ruan. 2007. Effect of onsite dietitian counseling on weight loss and lipid levels in an outpatient physician office. *American Journal of Cardiology* 100(1):73–75.

4

Transition to Community Care: Models and Opportunities

The focus of this session, moderated by Julie L. Locher, associate professor of medicine, Division of Gerontology, Geriatrics, and Palliative Care at the University of Alabama at Birmingham, was to identify models of transitioning to community care and opportunities for using these models to provide nutrition services. Presenters James A. Hester, Daniel J. Schoeps, Lori Gerhard, and Heather Keller each provided a discussion of specific models of transitional care and providing services in the community setting. The models discussed were the following:

- Centers for Medicare & Medicaid Services Innovation Center Models
  - Patient Care Model
  - Seamless Coordinated Care Model
  - Community and Population Health Models
- Veterans Directed Home- and Community-Based Services Program
- Canadian Models of Screening and Assessment in the Community
- Evergreen Action Nutrition Program in Canada

INNOVATIONS IN CARE TRANSITIONS: AN OVERVIEW

Presenter: James A. Hester

The Center for Medicare and Medicaid Innovation, known as the Innovation Center, is a new vehicle for improving care transitions said

James Hester, the Acting Director of the Population Health Models Group at the Innovation Center in the Centers for Medicare & Medicaid Services (CMS). The Innovation Center was created under the *Patient Protection and Affordable Care Act* Section 3021, to "test innovative payment and service delivery models to reduce program expenditures . . . while preserving or enhancing the quality of care" for those who get Medicare, Medicaid, or Children's Health Insurance Program benefits (P.L. 111-148 [May 2010]). The Innovation Center's mission is to be a trustworthy partner to identify, validate, and diffuse new models of care and payment that improve health and health care and reduce the total cost of care.

The Innovation Center: History and Organization

To begin, Hester posed the question, "Why should we innovate?" He suggested that innovation is a tool that can be used to decrease Medicaid and Medicare expenditures through improved care, thereby reducing the country's budget deficit. Hester also pointed to statistics that show 20 percent of Medicare recipients discharged from the hospital (11.8 million people) are readmitted within 30 days (Jencks et al., 2009). Many of those are readmitted due to preventable hospital-acquired conditions. He noted, however, the ultimate reason for innovation is the medical community's obligation to provide better health care.

The Innovation Center has $10 billion in funding through 2019 and has been given authority under the *Patient Protection and Affordable Care Act* that disables some of the constraints on Medicare demonstrations, particularly in regard to budget neutrality (P.L. 111-148, Sec. 2705). Hester explained that the budget neutrality requirement eliminated many promising innovations. If an innovation has been implemented, tested, and found to work effectively, "the Secretary can scale it up nationally" without having to return to Congress for new legislation.

The work of the Innovation Center is organized into three major model groups: (1) the Patient Care Model, (2) the Seamless Coordinated Care Model, and (3) Community and Population Health Models. The Patient Care Model focuses on what happens to a patient in a given episode of care at a given encounter. One initiative under this model is "bundled payments" in which multiple caregivers (e.g., from the surgeon to the postacute care facility) are reimbursed for treatment of a patient as a single episode with a single payment, thereby providing incentive for everyone to work together effectively. A second example of this model is Partnerships for Patients, a public-private partnership for a national patient safety campaign. (See below for further discussion of this initiative.)

The Seamless Coordinated Care Model involves coordinating care across the entire spectrum of the health community to improve health outcomes for patients. Hester stated that the existing health care system characteristically consists of "silos" within specific care settings resulting in rough transitions between the settings. Initiatives under the Seamless Coordinated Care Models that attempt to address this issue include the Multipayer Advanced Primary Care Practice demonstration project, the Pioneer Accountable Care Organizations (ACO) Model, and the Comprehensive Primary Care initiative.

The Community and Population Health Model explores how to improve the health of targeted populations with specific diseases, such as diabetes, as well as the well-being of communities as a whole. At-risk communities represent opportunities for improving health; and enhancing nutritional status is an aspect of health that can be pursued.

The Innovation Center solicits ideas for new models, selects the most promising, tests and evaluates the models, and finally disseminates the successful models. The measures of success are better health care experiences for patients, better health outcomes for populations, and reduced costs of care through improvement.

The Partnership for Patients Initiative mentioned above has two main goals: (1) a 40 percent reduction in preventable hospital-acquired conditions over 3 years and (2) a 20 percent reduction in 30-day readmissions in 3 years. Success in meeting these two goals could result in saving 60,000 lives and $35 billion in 3 years (CMS, 2011a). According to Hester, bipartisan support has been garnered due to the realization that improved patient outcomes through fewer preventable acquired conditions and fewer readmissions will result in large cost savings.

Care Transitions

Hester focused his discussion on the second goal (decreased readmissions) and noted that transition from one source of care to another is a period of high risk for communication failure, procedural errors, and unimplemented plans. He emphasized that the issue of poor care transitions and readmissions is concentrated in the most vulnerable populations—people with chronic conditions, organ system failure, and frailty. Hester indicated there is strong evidence demonstrating that hospital readmissions caused by flawed transitions can be significantly reduced.

The vision for successful care transitions, as outlined by Hester, is a care system in which each patient with complex needs has a plan that guides all care, moves with the patient across care settings, reflects the priorities of patient and family, and meets the needs of persons living with serious chronic conditions. Accomplishing that vision requires a combination of patient and caregiver engagement, patient-centered care plans, safe medication practices, and communication between the transferring and receiving providers. Importantly, the sending provider must maintain responsibility for the care of the patient until the receiving caregiver confirms the transfer and assumes responsibility, as opposed to a presumption that the transition went smoothly and the patient is well.

In order to achieve the goal of a 20 percent reduction in hospital readmissions, the Innovation Center estimated that a national network of 2,600 community-based care transition coalitions, partnering hospitals with community resources, would have to be built. Furthermore, a "roadmap" would be needed to help guide partnerships. The Partnership for Patients is building on evidence from research and pilot projects to support existing coalitions and encourage the formation of new ones. The Center provides data, technical support, money, consumer information, and training to support the partnerships and move the coalition forward in transition care.

The Innovation Center's strategy for the Partnership for Patients[1] program was to create very broad public-private partnerships; both commercial and philanthropic organizations have been involved. The aim was to have a portfolio of initiatives between communities and hospitals at various levels of development in providing transitional care. The Center established a simple hierarchy of these partnerships based on the level of their development, labeling them "walkers," "joggers," and "marathoners."

"Walkers" are the partnerships that are just beginning. Initiatives in place for "walkers" include the Quality Improvement Organizations (QIOs) and the Health Resources and Services Administration Patient Safety and Clinical Pharmacy Services Collaborative. QIOs are organizations staffed by health care professionals trained to review the medical care of beneficiaries and implement improvements in the quality of care. They provide technical assistance and other support to communities and hospitals in all 50 states, territories, and the District of Columbia. CMS enters into 3-year contracts, labeled as consecutively numbered Statements of Work (SOW), with the QIOs (CMS, 2011b). The QIO "9th SOW focused on improving the quality and safety of health care services to Medicare beneficiaries" (CMS, 2008). Lessons learned from the QIO 9th Scope of Work Care Transitions Theme include the importance of community collaboration, tailoring solutions to fit community priorities, including patients and families in decisions, and public outreach activities.

Hester said the main initiative for the "joggers" is the Community-Based Care Transitions Program (CCTP). CCTP, mandated by Section 3026 of the *Patient Protection and Affordable Care Act* (P.L. 111-148 [May 2010]), provides the opportunity for community-based organizations (CBOs) to partner with hospitals to improve transitions from hospitals

---

[1]Information on the Partnership for Patients campaign is available at http://www.healthcare. gov/center/programs/partnership/join/index.html.

to other care settings. The CCTP has $500 million available to support these partnerships and applications are now being accepted. The money is funneled through the CBOs, as opposed to the provider organizations, in order to strengthen the role of the CBO and strengthen the partnerships. The goals of the CCTP are to improve transitions of beneficiaries from the inpatient hospital setting to home or other care settings, reduce readmissions for high-risk beneficiaries, and document measurable savings to the Medicare program.

The final category of partnerships, the "marathoners," combines the seamless care initiatives of Bundled Payments for Care Improvement and ACOs.

Summary

Hester concluded by suggesting issues to be contemplated when considering care transitions:

- Examine how to build effective hospital-CBO partnerships and create an infrastructure of local CBOs where it does not exist.
- What are the key elements of a care plan? In particular, how can nutrition needs be incorporated into the care plan? Hester noted that needs should be identified; an effective entity for responding to those needs must be created that can recognize and seize the opportunity when the patient will be receptive to delivery of services.
- What payment policy changes are required to sustain better care transitions? Hester encouraged the audience to consider a sustainable payment and business model that can support services in the community over time.

VETERANS DIRECTED HOME- AND COMMUNITY-BASED SERVICES

Presenter: Daniel J. Schoeps and Lori Gerhard

Lori Gerhard, Director of the Office of Program Innovation and Demonstration for the U.S. Administration on Aging (AoA), opened the presentation by stating that AoA and the Veterans Health Administration (VHA) are interested in continuing to work together with registered dietitians and the nutrition community because nutrition is vital to helping people maintain their independence, health, and well-being and enabling them to be engaged in community life. Gerhard and Daniel J. Schoeps, Director of the Purchased Long-Term Care Group in the Office of Geriatrics and Extended Care at the Department of Veterans Affairs, presented on the role of the Veterans Directed Home- and Community-Based Services Program (VD-HCBS) in transitioning veterans to home- and community-based settings. The program has been under way for 3 years and lends itself to future models that can enable AoA and VHA to better serve people.

Historical Context and Development of the VD-HCBS Program

Schoeps provided a brief description of the Department of Veterans Affairs (VA), focusing on the VHA. The VHA has a $60 billion budget and 6 million veterans who use its services for health care in any given year. The VHA has 153 medical centers and 950 community-based outpatient clinics, 135 nursing homes, and 47 residential rehabilitation treatment centers. It is also affiliated with 107 medical schools, 55 dental schools, and 1,200 other schools for training and education purposes. Patient care, education, research, and backup to the Department of Defense in national emergencies are the four main missions of the VHA.

The partnership between VHA and AoA began over 35 years ago; however, the VD-HCBS has significantly changed the dynamic of that partnership. The organizations attempt to merge their expertise without duplicating activities. Veterans enrolled in VD-HCBS are in transition, such as those

- recently discharged from an inpatient hospital or nursing home setting,
- referred to VD-HCBS after an outpatient clinic visit,
- waiting to be admitted to a nursing home,
- recently admitted to a nursing home, or
- receiving traditional home care services but with insufficient quantity of support.

Veterans admitted into this program need to *choose* to participate because participation involves much work on their part. Potential clients for this program may be identified from the waiting list for a nursing home or as veterans who may be reconsidering their recent admission to a nursing home. Schoeps said that, through VD-HCBS, often clients can be offered more hours of care at home for the same cost of care they would receive through traditional services.

Gerhard continued by explaining the VHA was seeking a participant-directed model to engage the veteran in the design and delivery of his or her own care. At the same time, AoA was preparing to launch a demonstration grant program to reach older adults at risk of nursing home placement and of spend-down to Medicaid[2] to help them stay in the community. AoA was able to leverage that work to begin to develop VD-HCBS.

The research and programs that formed the basis to develop VD-HCBS included the following:

- National Long-Term Care Channeling Demonstration
- *Do Noninstitutional Long-Term Care Services Reduce Medicaid?* (Kaye et al., 2009)
- Chronic Care Model and Evidence-Based Care Transition Research
- Cash and Counseling Demonstration and Evaluation
- Stanford University Chronic Disease Self-Management Program Research

National Long-Term Care Channeling Demonstration

The Department of Health and Human Services (HHS) funded the National Long-Term Care Channeling Demonstration in 1980 as a model in 10 states to evaluate whether there was a way to change service delivery that would enable the government to serve the magnitude of people expected to need services in the future. The demonstration examined whether older adults who were enrolled in a program providing screening, assessment, care planning, service arrangements, follow-up, and reassessment could remain in the community, thereby avoiding placement in an institutional setting. The results showed no difference in the use of institutional care services, but other outcomes suggested further programming and evaluation were warranted. These outcomes included greater client satisfaction with life and the quality of care being received, as well as increased confidence in services being delivered and a reduction of unmet client needs (HHS ASPE, 1991). Gerhard indicated unmet needs are a risk factor for unnecessary admission to hospitals.

Do Noninstitutional Long-Term Care Services Reduce Medicaid?

The channeling demonstration gave way to the idea of the "woodwork effect." That is the concept that if access to home- and community-based services is expanded, the increased participation combined with continued nursing home expenditures raises the total cost of providing services to older adults for long-term care. However, more recent research done by Kaye et al. (2009) does not support this concept. Study results showed that, in the states that had robust home- and community-based service programs,

---

[2]The process of spending down one's assets to qualify for Medicaid. To qualify for Medicaid Spend-Down, a large part of one's income must be spent on medical care.

spending initially increased at a rapid pace because access to services was expanding. However, the increase was followed by a drop to a level of expenditure that was less than the original amount being spent, serving more people with fewer dollars. The results of this research began to inform AoA's and VHA's ongoing work.

Chronic Care Model and Evidence-Based Care Transition Research

The Chronic Care Model developed by Edward Wagner (see Figure 3-1) not only involves active patient participation, it also engages the larger community in the system. This model encourages coupling the strengths from the health care system and community resources to leverage opportunities to support the citizens in that community to have better health outcomes and quality of life (Wagner, 1998; Wagner et al., 2001). Evidence-based care transition research conducted by various scientists has shown how to form partnerships with people transitioning from hospital to home to facilitate, empower, and activate them to take control of their health and thrive in the community (Boult et al., 2008; Coleman, 2011; Counsell et al., 2006; Naylor et al., 2009).

Cash and Counseling Demonstration and Evaluation

The Cash and Counseling Demonstration and Evaluation, directed by Kevin Mahoney (Doty et al., 2007; Mahoney, 2005), was a concept tested in three states in which older adults received counseling and a flexible budget to personally obtain the care and services they most needed to remain in the community. Evaluation of this demonstration revealed higher satisfaction with care and services by both the individuals receiving care and their caregivers and reduced unmet needs of those requiring personal assistance. Medicaid personal care costs were somewhat higher, mainly because participants received more of the care they were authorized to receive. Gerhard explained that, under traditional delivery service systems, at times caregivers do not arrive to provide home care when scheduled, so the authorized care is not received. Under the Cash and Counseling Demonstration, participants were hiring family, friends, or neighbors and, thus, there was a higher reliability that services were delivered. The increased Medicaid personal care costs were partially offset by savings in institutional and other long-term care costs (NRCPDS, 2011).

Stanford University's Chronic Disease Self-Management Program

The last piece of research used was Stanford University's Chronic Disease Self-Management Program (CDSMP). This community-based program was designed to teach self-management skills to individuals with chronic disease conditions to improve health behaviors and outcomes (Lorig et al., 1999, 2001). HHS has contributed funding to this program since 2003, most recently under the American Recovery and Reinvestment Act, establishing CDSMPs for people with multiple chronic conditions in 45 states, the District of Columbia, and Puerto Rico.

Gerhard closed by noting that VD-HCBS is a partnership between administrative infrastructures. The goal for AoA is to assist the VA with rebalancing Long Term Services and Supports, which is currently spending about 80 percent of its budget on institutional care.

VD-HCBS Key Components

VD-HCBS provides veterans of all ages participant-directed HCBS options and empowers them to direct their own care. The goals of VD-HCBS are to increase the range of choices beyond traditional services and to provide the opportunity and ability for veterans to participate in design of services and planning of allocations for services. Veterans receive a participant-directed assessment performed in collaboration with an options counselor to develop a care plan. Together they manage a flexible service budget and decide what mix of goods and services will best meet their specific needs to live independently in the community. Each individual has his or her own unique situation and circumstances, so the veteran may hire and supervise their own service providers, including family or friends, and purchase items or other services to fill the gaps in care in a way that is most beneficial for the individual.

Another key component of VD-HCBS is the establishment of financial management services (FMS) entities throughout the country to assist the veterans with the management of their flexible service budget. The veteran is essentially an employer who must hire caregivers, negotiate rates for services and schedules, and provide a paycheck, which involves withholding taxes. The FMS entity assists with these tasks and issues fiscal reports on a monthly basis to the aging network engaged in the delivery of care to be able to ensure the fiscal accountability of the program.

Operations and Discovery

Schoeps reported that there are currently 33 operational VA Medical Center programs collaborating with 81 Area Agencies on Aging and Aging and Disability Resource Centers. Figure 4-1 indicates these locations as well as planned program sites.

Schoeps also highlighted discoveries made in the course of operating this program, saying it has been enlightening to see the types of services

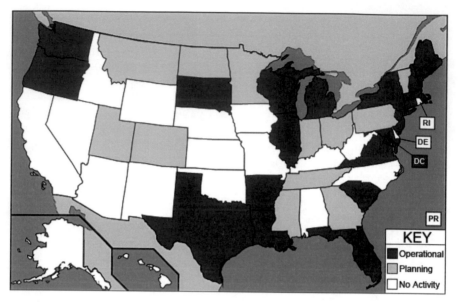

FIGURE 4-1 VD-HCBS operational and planned sites.
SOURCE: Schoeps and Gerhard, 2011.

the veterans are selecting and what they consider valuable. The majority choose to use their funds for personal care services, but other services have also been purchased. Schoeps gave an example of a young traumatic brain-injured veteran who needed to run. The vet identified someone to run with him and used his allotted money to pay for the service. The program will review invoices to learn what other new purchased services emerge. The VHA will also examine the relative cost of the VD-HCBS program as compared to the cost of traditional home care. Schoeps concluded by saying that the veterans-directed program has been well received by veterans and their families.

IMPROVING COMMUNITY NUTRITION CARE
FOR OLDER ADULTS IN CANADA

Presenter: Heather Keller

Transition care in Canada is somewhat fractured according to Heather Keller, a professor in the Department of Family Relations and Applied Nutrition at the University of Guelph in Ontario and a research scientist with the RBJ Schlegel-University of Waterloo Research Institute of Aging.

Although the Canadian Healthcare Act ensures that nationally all Canadian citizens receive universal health care, community health programs are very individualized and regionalized. Of the 34 million people in Canada, 14 percent of Canadians are over the age of 65 (Statistics Canada, 2011).

Keller discussed the role of nutrition screening in the context of a prevention model. In the community setting, screening is conducted on people who are asymptomatic in order to classify them as either likely or unlikely to have a specific disease (Morrison, 1992) or to identify nutritional risk (Posthauer et al., 1994). In an acute care setting, patients are already symptomatic and have significant risk factors.

Keller developed a process (see Figure 4-2) that examines the sectors of care around three levels of prevention. The process begins with primary prevention under the purview of public health units, which are funded by the ministries of health in each province, and primary care physicians. For example, dietitians may provide global messages about eating well that reach the entire population.

Secondary prevention includes early identification of asymptomatic people who are likely to experience health problems in attempts to prevent or delay progression of such problems. At this step in the process, screening is crucial and should be undertaken in the community. Secondary prevention efforts are carried out at social services agencies and wellness programs in the community, in addition to public health units and primary care offices. Primary care varies across Canadian provinces. For example, Ontario uses family health teams—dietitians, social workers, and kinesiologists located in doctors' offices conducting secondary prevention and treatment programs. Community services available to older adults in Canada at this level include meal programs, senior centers, transportation, and grocery delivery.

Tertiary prevention seeks to keep individuals who have already developed a chronic condition from declining in health, which Keller said is the goal of home care programs in Canada and nutrition programs for older adults in the United States. Tertiary prevention involves social service agencies, outpatient clinics, home care, and hospitals and includes typical medical model services, such as referrals to registered dietitians. The goal at the tertiary level is to keep older adults out of more expensive systems, such as nursing homes, which can actually contribute to further declines in their health.

Screening and Assessment

Keller posed the question, "How can screening promote secondary prevention?" Screening can identify the nutritional needs of older adults, thereby enabling services to be provided and appropriate referrals to be

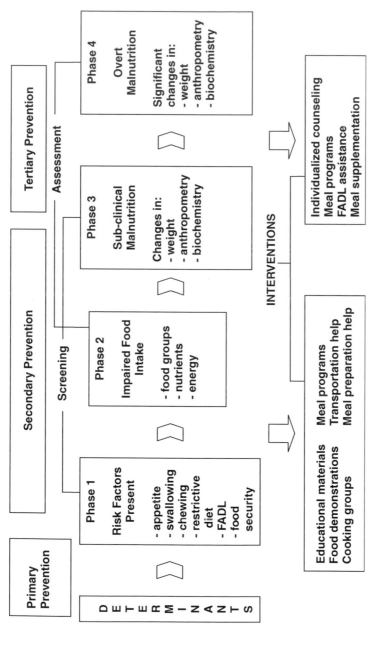

FIGURE 4-2 Screening and assessment across the continuum of care for older Canadians.

NOTE: FADL, food-related activities of daily living.

SOURCE: Adapted from H. H. Keller. 2007. Promoting food intake in older adults living in the community: A review. *Applied Psychology, Nutrition and Metabolism* 32(6):991–1000 © 2008 Canadian Science Publishing or its licensors. Reproduced with permission.

made to other community programs. It can also raise awareness of nutrition and health risks for the older adults and their families, prompting behavior change.

Screening and assessment can be thought of as overlapping activities that occur across four phases which make up a continuum of malnutrition (Figure 4-2). Initially, the health care professional reviews risk factors that may contribute to impaired food intake, such as poor appetite. The next phase involves progression of risk factors so that food intake is impaired, while the third phase is the presence of subclinical malnutrition identified by either screening or assessment as identified by changes in anthropometric and biochemical measurements. Significant anthropometric, biochemical, and functional changes as seen in phase 4 indicate overt malnutrition, which is the end state assessed only with a comprehensive assessment.

Interventions that may be implemented as a result of screening in phases 1 and 2 would center on food-related activities of daily living, such as grocery shopping, cooking, meal delivery, meal preparation, and transportation. Assessment during the later phases would require additional higher-end interventions, including individualized counseling, meal programs, and meal supplementation.

Keller described SCREEN, a paper-and-pencil nutrition risk tool used to evaluate older adults in the community. SCREEN stands for Seniors in the Community: Risk Evaluation for Eating and Nutrition and can be self-administered or completed by an interviewer. SCREEN was validated against the criterion of a dietitian's assessment of nutritional risk and demonstrated test-retest reliability and an intermodal and inter-rater reliability. SCREEN is not only a tool, but a screening program that includes a referral process to services and educational needs based on identified risk items (Keller, 2007; Keller et al., 2006a).

Keller described an ethical screening process involving identification of an individual at risk through initial screening, followed by a referral to a physician or dietitian for nutritional assessment and treatment if necessary. The individual may also be referred to other professionals and services, such as a social worker or family counselor. Subsequently, since a new program of care was implemented, the client restarts the cycle of rescreening to be monitored continuously.

She then reviewed a screening demonstration project conducted with 1,200 older adults in five diverse communities in Canada. A referral system was developed to link the adults with services in their communities. For example, if they were identified as high risk at a Meals On Wheels Program, they could be referred to receive more meals, a congregate dining program, or a dietitian. Sixty percent of those identified as "at risk" refused referrals because they either felt their current services were sufficient or did not feel nutrition was a priority for them at that point. Of those referred, 62 percent were referred to a dietitian but faced barriers related to long waiting times, cost, access, and doctors unwilling to make the necessary referral. Twenty-three percent of referrals were to the Meals On Wheels program, but reported barriers to participation included cost and dislike of the food (Keller et al., 2007).

Keller mentioned a small pilot study illustrating that behavior and knowledge can be changed through provision of an education pamphlet and administration of a screening tool alone (Southgate et al., 2010), suggesting that self-management of screening might be a consideration.

Over the past year, Keller has been collaborating with dietitians in Canada to develop an Internet version of SCREEN (www.eatrightontario.ca/escreen/) for older adults. It is a self-management tool, allowing older adults to assess their own nutritional risk. The screening tool guides the individual to credible educational resources and activities that can assist in changing his or her behavior.

Other Research

A study being conducted by the Canadian Malnutrition Task Force is examining the prevalence of malnutrition upon admission to and discharge from the hospital; the nutrition process during the hospital stay; and outcomes at 30 days, including readmission and mortality. To date, 10 hospitals are collecting data and expect to have studied 500 patients by the end of the year; the goal is 1,000 patients. Using Subjective Global Assessment and albumin status, preliminary data from 160 patients indicate that 45 percent of people admitted were malnourished. At discharge, although the percentage is reduced, 35 percent are still in a malnourished state. Keller surmised that these data are indicative of the malnutrition that occurs in the community and demonstrate that Canada and the United States experience the same problems with transitional care.

In another study, conducted by Keller and McKenzie (2003), vulnerable older adults across Canada who participated in home care and Meals On Wheels were surveyed to determine their nutrition-related risk factors. Results are shown in Table 4-1.

Community Services in Canada

Keller noted that Canada does not have an elder nutrition program comparable to that of the AoA. She explained this may be in part because the base-level annual income for persons over the age of 65 in Canada is $15,000 and perhaps this supports free medical care, medications, and access to home care if eligibility criteria are met. However, Keller explained that home care is not part of the act in which national health care is pro-

TABLE 4-1 Percent of Older Canadians Reporting Nutrition-Related Risk Factors

Nutrition-Related Risk Factor	Percent of Participants Reporting Risk Factor
Difficulty shopping	89
Low fruit and vegetable intake	48
Restricts food intake	45
Difficulty cooking	42
Difficulty chewing	34.6
Weight change	33
Poor appetite	28
Difficulty swallowing	22.9
Weight loss	22

SOURCE: Keller and McKenzie, 2003.

vided to every citizen in Canada. It is considered an extended service, and services can vary among provinces or even communities within a province.

The Inter-RAI Home Care Assessment System[3] is used in several provinces to screen for advanced nutrition problems, such as unintended weight loss of 5 percent in 30 days, cachexia, or enteral nutrition. Keller indicated that relatively few people (e.g., < 20 percent) in home care trigger the need for a dietitian service using this assessment, although Keller believes that in reality many of participants are malnourished. In Keller's opinion, the use of this tool does not adequately identify those people with unmet nutritional needs whose health may be improved with nutrition services that can prevent further decline.

In general throughout Canada, meal programs are arranged through referral to social service agencies, long-term care hospitals, Red Cross programs, or similar organizations. Government funding for meal programs is nonexistent, apart from a small amount of subsidies for which organizations must apply. Meal services are primarily financially supported by philanthropic programs or fee-for-service payments (fees vary by location) and are delivered by volunteers. Home aides also prepare meals and assist with basic activities, but the services provided vary by province.

The Evergreen Action Nutrition Program is an example of a successful community education and secondary prevention program in Canada. It was developed to provide some of the services and information that seniors want—food workshops, cooking classes for older men, and information

---

[3]A person-centered assessment system, focusing on the person's functioning and quality of life by assessing needs, strengths, and preferences, that informs and guides comprehensive care and service planning in community-based settings (http://www.interrai.org/section/view/?fnode=15).

to support behavioral changes to improve dietary intake. The program was funded for 3 years at $70,000 through a research grant. Through this program fruit and vegetable intake improved, men learned new cooking skills, 94 percent of participants reported increased nutrition knowledge, and 50 percent of participants reported increased pleasure from eating (Keller et al., 2004, 2005, 2006b). In the diabetes support groups, 50 percent of participants changed their diet, 56 percent lost excess weight, and 50 percent had lower blood sugars (Keller, unpublished data).

Summary

Keller summarized the highlights of her presentation, noting that the nutrition problems in Canada are consistent with those in the United States. She stated that older adults want to improve their nutrition, are motivated to do so, and can implement secondary prevention interventions. Although screening programs can lead to secondary prevention and be models for producing linkages to services in the community, there is inadequate funding for secondary prevention in Canada. Finally, there is a place for self-management of nutrition needs which requires support in Canada.

Keller suggested that research priorities include the following:

- Demonstrating the effectiveness of nutrition screening programs in the community
- Identifying best practices for transition to the community from the hospital and answering questions such as "What forms of communication are needed between sectors?"
- Exploring the use of a social care model versus a medical need model for home care services

DISCUSSION

Moderator: Julie Locher

The discussion focused on nutrition in transitional care and patient-directed care of the frail.

Nutrition in Transitional Care

Gordon Jensen asked about concrete plans for transitional care—specifically related to nutrition concerns—from acute care, subacute care, or chronic care back home to independent living for people at high risk of readmission. Locher proposed that a significant barrier to providing nutrition services during transitional care is reimbursement for registered dietitians (RDs) to provide such services in the community setting. Although hospitals and home health care agencies are required to have RDs on staff, in the community setting the mechanism for an RD to independently request reimbursement is cumbersome and the amount so minimal it is not to the dietitian's benefit to seek reimbursement. Hester pointed to the Section 3026 Community-Based Care Transition Program as an ideal vehicle for a local community organization in partnership with the hospital to design a nutrition intervention. Flexibility is given to the community to determine priorities in needed services. A proposal, which includes nutrition services requiring the support of an RD, could be developed and then the payment model would be included. Therefore, he suggested the goal should be to raise the awareness of the communities that nutrition needs to be a key part of transition care when developing specific proposals. He continued by saying to the extent that the focus is on a patient-centered model, noting the importance of listening to the patients and patient-driven goals as Eric Coleman discussed, the task is to determine how to increase patients' awareness of their nutritional needs in order to make nutrition services a priority among their requests.

Gerhard suggested that, as the consumer gets more involved, RDs should consider ways to package their services in a way that consumers with funds could purchase them.

Nancy Wellman asked whether a list of available services is provided through CMS or the VD-HCBS and, if so, is nutrition one of the services listed? Schoeps replied that the VD-HCBS does have a list of services that includes nutrition. Hester stated that Section 3026 does not offer a list of potential services, as it is left to the community to determine the appropriate mix of services to provide based on a root-cause analysis of the patients in their community and then develop a proposal. It is not a prescriptive program, but provides flexibility to meet individual community needs.

Patient-Directed Care of the Frail

A participant suggested that patient-directed care is not realistic for the frail older adult, since the responsibilities would be more than such a person is able to manage and caregivers are already overwhelmed. Gerhard reported that people with disabilities have expressed the belief that they know best how to train caregivers to provide care to them. Schoeps said the majority of veterans enrolled in VD-HCBS are older persons, many of whom choose to have a representative make the day-to-day decisions (e.g., a spouse). Additionally, the financial management services entities complete much of the paperwork involved in employing a caregiver.

Connie Bales suggested that nutrition services are about changing behaviors, which is different than assisting with physical needs. She questioned, "How do we let the patient decide what's good for them when they don't know [what that is]?" Keller responded that screening can be a very effective tool in raising self-awareness of health-related issues. She proposed the self-directed model can come with screening, because sometimes people do not know what their needs are until confronted with a screening tool that identifies an issue that indicates a health risk. For example, it may be that if the person has a poor appetite, he or she may realize that is not normal, but until they have a conversation with a health care provider about this risk and learn that there are services available (e.g., congregate dining) that may help, they are not typically going to see the need for the service.

REFERENCES

Boult, C., L. Karm, and C. Groves. 2008. Improving chronic care: The "guided care" model. *The Permanente Journal* 12(1):50–54.

CMS (Centers for Medicare & Medicaid Services). 2008. *CMS Awards Contracts for Quality Improvement Organizations' 9th Statement of Work*. https://www.cms.gov/qualityimprovementorgs/downloads/9thsowannouncement080508.pdf (accessed November 3, 2011).

CMS. 2011a. *Partnership for Patients*. http://innovations.cms.gov/areas-of-focus/patient-care-models/partnerships-for-patients/ (accessed November 3, 2011).

CMS. 2011b. *Quality Improvement Organizations*. https://www.cms.gov/qualityimprovementorgs/ (accessed November 3, 2011).

Coleman, E. A. 2011. *The Care Transitions Program®*. http://www.caretransitions.org/ (accessed December 12, 2011).

Counsell, S. R., C. M. Callahan, A. B. Buttar, D. O. Clark, and K. I. Frank. 2006. Geriatric Resources for Assessment and Care of Elders (GRACE): A new model of primary care for low-income seniors. *Journal of the American Geriatrics Society* 54(7):1136–1141.

Doty, P., K. J. Mahoney, and L. Simon-Rusinowitz. 2007. Designing the Cash and Counseling Demonstration and Evaluation. *Health Services Research* 42(1 Pt II):378–396.

HHS ASPE (U.S. Department of Health and Human Services Office for the Assistant Secretary for Planning and Evaluation). 1991. *National Long-Term Care Channeling Demonstration: Summary of Demonstration and Reports*. Washington, DC: HHS ASPE. http://aspe.hhs.gov/daltcp/reports/chansum.pdf (accessed December 22, 2011).

Jencks, S. F., M. V. Williams, and E. A. Coleman. 2009. Rehospitalizations among patients in the Medicare Fee-for-Service Program. *New England Journal of Medicine* 360(14):1418–1428.

Kaye, H. S., M. P. LaPlante, and C. Harrington. 2009. Do noninstitutional long-term care services reduce Medicaid spending? *Health Affairs* 28(1):262–272.

Keller, H. H. 2007. Promoting food intake in older adults living in the community: A review. *Applied Physiology, Nutrition and Metabolism* 32(6):991–1000.

Keller, H. H., and J. D. McKenzie. 2003. Nutritional risk: In vulnerable community-living seniors. *Canadian Journal of Dietetic Practice and Research* 64(4):195–201.

Keller, H. H., A. Gibbs, S. Wong, P. D. Vanderkooy, and M. Hedley. 2004. Men can cook! Development, implementation, and evaluation of a senior men's cooking group. *Journal of Nutrition for the Elderly* 24(1):71–87.

Keller, H. H., M. R. Hedley, T. Hadley, S. Wong, and P. D. Vanderkooy. 2005. Food workshops, nutrition education, and older adults: A process evaluation. *Journal of Nutrition
for the Elderly* 24(3):5–23.

Keller, H. H., B. Brockest, and H. Haresign. 2006a. Building capacity for nutrition risk screening. *Nutrition Today* 11(1):161–170.

Keller, H. H., M. R. Hedley, S. S. L. Wong, P. Vanderkooy, J. Tindale, and J. Norris. 2006b.
Community organized food and nutrition education: Participation, attitudes and nutritional risk in seniors. *Journal of Nutrition, Health and Aging* 10(1):15–20.

Keller, H. H., H. Haresign, and B. Brockest. 2007. Process evaluation of Bringing Nutrition Screening to Seniors in Canada (BNSS). *Canadian Journal of Dietetic Practice and
Research* 68(2):86–91.

Lorig, K. R., D. S. Sobel, A. L. Stewart, B. W. Brown Jr., A. Bandura, P. Ritter, V. M. Gonzalez,
D. D. Laurent, and H. R. Holman. 1999. Evidence suggesting that a chronic disease
self-management program can improve health status while reducing hospitalization a
randomized trial. *Medical Care* 37(1):5–14.

Lorig, K. R., P. Ritter, A. L. Stewart, D. S. Sobel, B. W. Brown Jr., A. Bandura, V. M.
Gonzalez, D. D. Laurent, and H. R. Holman. 2001. Chronic disease self-management
program: 2-year health status and health care utilization outcomes. *Medical Care*
39(11):1217–1223.

Mahoney, K. J. 2005. *Cash & Counseling: Congressional Briefing.* http://www.allhealth.org/
briefingmaterials/Mahoney-194.pdf (accessed November 30, 2011).

Morrison, A. S. 1992. Screening in chronic disease. In *Monographs in Epidemiology and
Biostatistics,* 2nd ed. New York: Oxford University Press.

Naylor, M. D., P. H. Feldman, S. Keating, M. J. Koren, E. T. Kurtzman, M. C. MacCoy, and
R. Krakauer. 2009. Translating research into practice: Transitional care for older adults.
Journal of Evaluation in Clinical Practice 15(6):1164–1170.

NRCPDS (National Resource Center for Participant-Driven Services). 2011. *Cash & Counseling.* http://www.bc.edu/schools/gssw/nrcpds/cash_and_counseling.html (accessed November 30, 2011).

Posthauer, M. E., B. Dorse, R. A. Foiles, S. Escott-Stump, L. Lysen, and L. Balogun. 1994.
Identifying patients at risk: ADA's definitions for nutrition screening and nutrition assessment. *Journal of the American Dietetic Association* 94(8):838–839.

Schoeps, D. J., and L. Gerhard. 2011. *The Veterans Directed Home & Community Based
Services (VD-HCBS) Program.* Presented at the Institute of Medicine Workshop on Nutrition and Healthy Aging in the Community. Washington, DC, October 5–6.

Southgate, K. M., H. H. Keller, and H. D. Reimer. 2010. Determining knowledge and behaviour change: After nutrition screening among older adults. *Canadian Journal of Dietetic
Practice and Research* 71(3):128–133.

Statistics Canada. 2011. *Canada's Population Estimates: Age and Sex.* http://www.statcan.
gc.ca/daily-quotidien/110928/dq110928a-eng.htm (accessed November 28, 2011).

Wagner, E. H. 1998. Chronic disease management: What will it take to improve care for
chronic illness? *Effective Clinical Practice* 1(1):2–4.

Wagner, E. H., B. T. Austin, C. Davis, M. Hindmarsh, J. Schaefer, and A. Bonomi. 2001.
Improving chronic illness care: Translating evidence into action. *Health Affairs*
20(6):64–78.

5

Successful Intervention Models in the Community Setting

This session focused on the successes and challenges of developing practical interventions that address the nutrition needs of older adults in the community. Douglas Paddon-Jones, associate professor at the University of Texas Medical Branch and the session moderator, noted that the strength of this session was the practitioner-based approaches presented by speakers with expertise in nursing, physical therapy, and gerontology. The interventions that were discussed include the following:

- Community telephonic interventions
  — Vision is Precious Program
  — Improving Diabetes Outcome Study
- The Diabetes Prevention Program
- Medical nutrition therapy
  — Dietary Approaches to Stop Hypertension (DASH) Diet
- Nutrition interventions for frailty and sarcopenia
- Eat Better, Move More program

DIABETES SELF-MANAGEMENT SUPPORT IN THE COMMUNITY: HEALTHY EATING CONSIDERATIONS

Presenter: Elizabeth A. Walker

Elizabeth Walker, professor of medicine, and epidemiology and population health at Albert Einstein College of Medicine, described two theoretical approaches used in diabetes self-management interventions. The first, community telephonic interventions, falls under the community category of Ed Wagner's Chronic Care Model (see Chapter 3, Figure 3-1). The goal of these interventions is to produce informed and active patients who interact productively with their health care teams to improve outcomes (Wagner, 1998; Wagner et al., 2001). The second approach she discussed, the social-ecological model, is used to inform the development of interventions that address individual behavior and influences within their environment of family, community, culture, and policy issues (Fisher et al., 2002; Stokels, 1996).

Walker suggested that diabetes self-management interventions include methods for addressing the American Association of Diabetes Educators' seven self-care behaviors:

1.   healthy eating
2.   being active
3.   monitoring
4.   taking medication
5.   problem solving
6.   healthy coping
7.   reducing risks

Since types 1 and 2 diabetes are chronic conditions, Walker suggested that psychosocial interventions should focus on treatment adherence through motivating behavior change and emotional support. These interventions include goal setting, problem solving, maintenance strategies, continuing support, and treatment of distress and psychiatric disorders such as depression. In addition, the interventions should include some form of activation, such as coaching or empowerment, and be tailored to meet the individual's needs (Peyrot and Rubin, 2007).

Telephonic Interventions

A telephonic intervention can be used as a stand-alone intervention, or as part of a multicomponent intervention such as one that includes face-to-face interviews. Depending on available funding, the intervention can consist of an automated voice message, text message (personalized or not), or person-to-person conversation. Walker noted that the interventions she developed involve person-to-person conversations because she and her researchers have not determined appropriate wording for an automated voice or text message that would effectively improve motivation or self-care behaviors. Telephonic interventions can be used multiple ways within an intervention, such as focusing on improving participants' glycemic control and medication adherence or as a supplement to a diabetes education program during the maintenance phase. Regardless of how they are used, interventions should be tailored to meet the needs of the target population, to take into account costs and benefits, and, if necessary, to be scalable and translatable (Schechter et al., 2008; Walker et al., 2008).

The Vision is Precious Program was a telephonic intervention used to promote diabetic retinopathy screening within 6 months among low-income minority adults who had not had a dilated eye exam in over a year. It resulted in a 74 percent increase in the rate of screening in the intervention group as compared to the control group that received a printed booklet in the mail (Walker et al., 2008). Walker pointed out that this intervention was for a single behavior, and it is more difficult for interventions to produce the multiple behavior changes needed to improve diabetes control.

Improving Diabetes Outcome Study

The Improving Diabetes Outcome Study was a randomized controlled trial focused on adults 30 years and older who were prescribed oral diabetes medication, had HbA_{1c} levels at or below 7.5 percent, were members or spouses of the health care workers labor union, and had less than optimal medication adherence. The aims of the study are listed in Box 5-1.

The social cognitive theory was used to emphasize self-efficacy and tailor the intervention to the participants' readiness to change stage (Bandura, 1986). Participants in the intervention group could receive up to 10 phone calls from a health educator over 12 months and discussed a diabetes-related behavior of the participant's choosing during those calls.

BOX 5-1
Specific Aims of the *Improving Diabetes Outcome Study*

- Aim 1: A tailored telephone intervention compared to a standard print (active control) intervention will significantly improve glycemic control measured by HbA_{1c}.

- Aim 2: A tailored telephone intervention . . . will significantly improve medication adherence and lifestyle behaviors.

- Aim 3: To describe characteristics of those who benefit most from the telephonic intervention.

- Aim 4: To evaluate costs of the intervention.

The active control group received printed self-management materials. The majority of participants in both groups were female (67 percent), non-Hispanic black (61.6 percent), and foreign-born (76.8 percent), and the average body mass index was 31.2 (obese) (Walker et al., 2011).

Participants in the intervention group had significant improvements in their HbA_{1c} levels, a reduction of 0.36 percent difference from the active control group (see Figure 5-1). Adjusted multivariate analysis of the HbA_{1c} levels showed that older age, lower income, and higher baseline HbA_{1c} were independently associated with improved HbA_{1c}. While the third finding was not surprising because higher levels are somewhat easier to improve, Walker did note that the first two results suggest that the intervention was well tailored to this group.

Participants received, on average, eight calls totaling about 109 minutes over 12 months. Calls ranged in length from 2 to 35 minutes, with a mean length of less than 15 minutes. Results indicated that there was an improvement in HbA_{1c} among those people who received 6 phone calls or more; however, there was not a linear relationship between number of phone calls and amount of HbA_{1c} improvement (Walker et al., 2011).

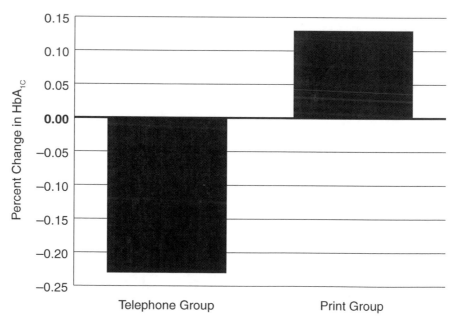

FIGURE 5-1 Change in HbA_{1c} baseline to end of study.
SOURCE: Walker et al., 2011.

Associations between participation in self-care activities (from the Summary of Diabetes Self-Care Activities [Toobert and Glasgow, 1994]) and participation in the intervention were analyzed. While there were associations between several activities and the intervention (e.g., thinking about healthy eating), only two activities were significantly associated with the telephone intervention: (1) the number of days per week following a healthy eating plan and (2) exercising for 30 minutes or more. However, none of the activities was significantly associated with improved HbA_{1c} levels (Walker et al., 2011). Walker concluded that "small improvements in self-care activities may add up to a meaningful HbA_{1c} improvement."

The Diabetes Prevention Program

The Diabetes Prevention Program (DPP) was a randomized clinical trial aimed at preventing type 2 diabetes in high-risk people. Study participants were randomized into one of three groups: (1) intensive lifestyle (Wylie-Rosett and Delahanty, 2002), (2) metformin, or (3) placebo. On average, the lifestyle changes and metformin groups resulted in 58 and 31 percent reductions of risk, respectively (Knowler et al., 2002). In the 60 years and older group, which comprised about 20 percent of the total study population, lifestyle changes produced a 70 percent reduction of risk. As compared to the other age groups, this age group experienced the most weight loss, the greatest reduction in waist circumference, the most recreational activity per week, and the most people who met their weight loss and exercise goals (Crandall et al., 2006; Diabetes Prevention Program Research Group, 2009; Wing, 2004). As summarized by Walker, "lifestyle modifications can prevent diabetes or delay diabetes in high-risk older people" and reduce cardiovascular risk and urinary incontinence (Brown et al., 2006). Furthermore, people preferred the lifestyle modifications to taking the medication (Crandall et al., 2006; Diabetes Prevention Program Research Group, 2009; Wing, 2004).

Closing Comments

Lower cost interventions can be effective at addressing health behaviors provided they are tailored to the needs of the target population. Diabetes self-management or prevention interventions, including those conducted over the telephone, can result in improved medication adherence, behavior change, weight loss, reduced glucose intolerance, and lowered diabetes risk if the intervention focuses on behaviors selected by the participants. Since self-management interventions may address various diabetes self-care behaviors, including healthy eating and medication, experts in diverse fields should be involved as participants decide what behavior they would like to change.

NUTRITION INTERVENTION FOR CARDIOVASCULAR DISEASE: HOME-DELIVERED MEDICAL NUTRITION THERAPY AND DASH MEALS

Presenter: Jennifer L. Troyer

Jennifer L. Troyer, associate professor and chair of the Department of Economics at the University of North Carolina at Charlotte, discussed nutrition interventions she conducted with older adults. She described the results of providing medical nutrition therapy (MNT) and therapeutic meals to older adults with cardiovascular disease in their homes, including data on adherence to a modified diet, changes in dietary knowledge, health outcomes, and cost effectiveness.

Medical Nutrition Therapy

The Institute of Medicine recommended MNT to promote the health of older adults with chronic illnesses (IOM, 2000). MNT is a multisession intervention though which a registered dietitian (RD) determines the type and frequency of nutrition care appropriate for the individual's medical condition. The RD conducts a lifestyle assessment and helps the individual develop goals that are revisited in future sessions (Gehling, 2011; Michael, 2001; Rezabek, 2001). It is "more intensive, diagnosis-specific, and behavior-oriented than traditional nutrition counseling," said Troyer.

The American Dietetic Association recommends MNT for people with cardiovascular disease as the initial intervention for people with hypertension and hyperlipidemia (McCaffree, 2003) based on evidence that it is the best option for treatment of hyperlipidemia (Baron, 2005) and has been found to lower serum cholesterol and LDL levels among people with hypertension (Delahanty et al., 2001, 2002; Lim et al., 2008; Sikand et al., 2000). In 2000, Congress authorized RDs as eligible providers of MNT under Medicare, but only for renal disease and diabetes because of the strong effectiveness data available for those conditions (Franz et al., 2008). There is some evidence that MNT is a cost-effective way to reduce serum cholesterol levels, but not elevated blood pressure. However, these randomized clinical trials were not restricted to older adults and did not include data on general medical costs that may be affected by MNT; rather they only considered costs of conducting the interventions (Pavlovich et al., 2004).

Therapeutic Meals: The DASH Diet

Therapeutic meals are "designed in accordance with dietary guidance in an effort to assist in disease management through dietary modification," said Troyer. The therapeutic meals provided to participants in this intervention were designed based on the Dietary Approaches to Stop Hypertension (DASH) diet. The DASH diet repeatedly has been found as an effective way to reduce blood pressure through lifestyle and diet changes. It is designed to reduce intake of saturated fat, total fat, sodium, and cholesterol; increase intakes of fruits and vegetables; and increase consumption of potassium, calcium, magnesium, fiber, and protein (Appel et al., 1997; Blumenthal et al., 2010; Dickinson et al., 2006; Elmer et al., 2006; Lin et al., 2007; Sacks et al., 2001).

Clinical Trial

This intervention considered the effects of MNT and therapeutic meals on changes in adherence to the DASH diet and changes in dietary knowledge among community-dwelling adults ages 60 years and older diagnosed with high cholesterol, high blood pressure, or both. Since Medicare funds MNT for individuals with diabetes or renal disease, those individuals along with those that had recent surgery or adverse health conditions were excluded from the study. Participants were randomized into one of four groups, as shown in Figure 5-2.

The "literature" group received brochures containing information on how to handle their high blood pressure or high cholesterol. The "meals" and "MNT and meals" groups received frozen meals that conformed to Administration on Aging (AoA) requirements that meals provide one-third of participants' Dietary Reference Intakes and adhere to the *Dietary Guidelines for Americans*. In addition they received milk, calcium-fortified orange

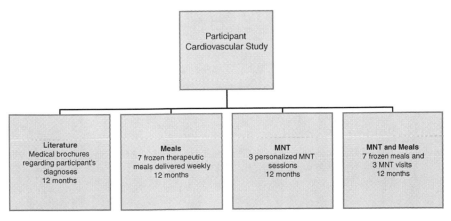

FIGURE 5-2 Clinical trial design.
SOURCE: Troyer, 2011.

juice, and some shelf-stable products. The two groups receiving MNT were provided therapy in their homes by an RD who also assessed participants' food and cooking situation and provided MNT to caregivers, if applicable.

Data were collected at baseline, 6 months, and 12 months on 298 participants. Study participants were primarily white (61 percent), women (83 percent), and had incomes above the poverty line (52 percent had incomes greater than 165 percent of the poverty level). Twenty-eight percent had hypertension, 20 percent had hyperlipidemia, 54 percent had both hypertension and hyperlipidemia, and 80 percent were taking medication to manage their hypertension or hyperlipidemia. The data were analyzed to answer three questions:

1. *Do home-delivered DASH meals change adherence to a DASH diet?* The DASH diet includes nine dietary recommendations for intake of protein, total fat, saturated fat, cholesterol, fiber, magnesium, calcium, potassium, and sodium. Participants were scored as "DASH accordant" and "intermediate DASH accordant" based on the number of nutrient targets they reached or partially reached. Between baseline and 6 months, there was a significant increase in the percentage of participants who adhered to a DASH diet; recipients of DASH meals had a 20-percentage-point-higher probability of being intermediate DASH accordant at 6 months than those who did not receive the meals, with higher gains among whites and higher-income individuals. Nonwhite meal recipients had significant reductions in cholesterol intake and significant gains in intermediate DASH scores and fiber intake as compared to nonwhites who did not receive the meals (Troyer et al., 2010a). From baseline to 12 months there was less change, which Troyer described as participants "losing a little bit of speed at the end of the study."

2. *Does home-delivered MNT affect dietary knowledge and dietary change?* Participants in the literature-only or MNT-only groups were administered a 20-question survey on dietary knowledge. While there was no significant change in dietary knowledge from baseline to 6 months, MNT recipients had a 1.88 point (out of 20) increase from baseline to 12 months. The effects of MNT on knowledge gain were higher for whites, those not living alone, those with less than a high school diploma, and those with income below the poverty level. Increases in dietary knowledge produced few significant results and no positive change in adherence to a DASH diet. Troyer posited reasons for the results may have been poor delivery, reluctance of people to change, or inability to translate knowledge into behavior change (Racine et al., 2011).

3. *Are home-delivered MNT and DASH meals cost-effective?* Cost data were collected on MNT administration; therapeutic meal production and delivery; and participant-level medical costs, pharmaceuticals, and personal assistance costs. In addition, quantity and quality of life gained were measured in quality-adjusted life years (QALYs). Troyer stated that the question to be answered is "what does it cost [society] in terms of this intervention to generate a year of life at full health?" If society is willing to pay $109,000 for one QALY (Braithwaite et al., 2008), then the probability that the therapeutic meals program is cost-effective is 95 percent, that MNT is cost-effective is 90 percent, and that therapeutic meals plus MNT is cost-effective is less than 50 percent (Troyer et al., 2010b).

Closing Remarks

Providing home-delivered DASH meals to older adults with cardiovascular disease is likely to change adherence to a DASH diet. Therefore, Troyer suggests further research to explore the differential effects of meals by recipient's income level and to determine if meal customization for those with multiple conditions is feasible and cost-effective. Further research is needed to review the relationship between dietary knowledge and dietary change, to determine the role that food insecurity plays in dietary change, and to conduct a cost-benefit analysis of home-delivered MNT.

Troyer noted that cost-effectiveness results suggest that Medicare should consider paying for MNT for cardiovascular disease because costs would be less than suggested in the study if MNT were provided in a "real-world" setting; over 80 percent of study participants were taking medication; the study included a small dose of MNT; and data were collected on participants that dropped out of the study yet, despite these factors that would bias the findings toward no positive results, still obtained positive results.

NUTRITION INTERVENTIONS FOR FRAILTY AND SARCOPENIA

Presenter: Elena Volpi

The cycle of frailty, to which chronic undernutrition and sarcopenia contribute, can lead to reductions in strength and power and increased risk of falls and injuries which may lead to physical dependence. Elena Volpi, professor of internal medicine–geriatrics at the University of Texas Medical Branch, presented research illustrating the importance of protein intake and intake patterns in determining the rates of muscle protein synthesis and anabolism and their potential role in the prevention of muscle loss in older adults.

Muscle Protein Synthesis

Sarcopenia is the "universal, progressive and involuntary decline in lean body mass and function associated with aging, primarily due to loss of skeletal muscle" (Roubenoff and Castaneda, 2001), leading to loss of strength and power. Maintaining muscle mass and strength is important for older adults because strength is associated with mortality; in the Health Aging and Body Composition (ABC) study, older adults with initially greater strength were more likely to be alive after an average 5-year follow-up than those with initially lower strength (Newman et al., 2006). Another paper from the Health ABC group shows that habitual protein intake also predicted muscle loss; older persons with the highest protein intake lost the least amount of muscle mass (Houston et al., 2008).

The process by which insulin stimulates muscle protein synthesis during a meal is impaired in older adults (Volpi et al., 2000). This can be considered a true insulin resistance, as larger doses of insulin can stimulate protein synthesis in healthy older adults (Fujita et al., 2009; Rasmussen et al., 2006). Since there is no other inactive, immediately accessible reservoir for protein, the protein that is not synthesized into muscle in older adults is converted to fat or oxidized, further contributing to sarcopenia, obesity, and loss of function.

This reduced protein synthesis response in older adults can be normalized if a vasodilator is administered along with the increased insulin (Timmerman et al., 2010a). Vasodilation seems to be a fundamental regulator of the response of muscle protein synthesis to insulin in younger persons (Timmerman et al., 2010b). "The good news is that you don't need a drug to get [vasodilation in older adults]," said Volpi, "aerobic exercise can do that as well." Preliminary data from Timmerman and colleagues also suggest that aerobic exercise can improve the response of muscle protein synthesis to a meal in older adults. "So," Volpi summarized, "physical activity is fundamental, it looks like, for maintenance of the anabolic stimulation of muscle protein synthesis by a meal."

Protein Intake to Maximize Muscle Protein Synthesis

How much protein should older adults consume to maximize muscle protein synthesis? Katsanos and colleagues (2006) studied the relationship between various amounts of leucine, the amino acid that stimulates protein synthesis in muscle, and changes in protein synthesis. An amount of 1.7 g of leucine increased protein synthesis by 30 percent in young adults but produced no change in that of older adults. Both the young and older adults showed about a 50 percent increase in synthesis when given 2.8 and 3.2 g of leucine, leading researchers to conclude that a dose of about 2.8 g of leucine maximally stimulates muscle protein synthesis during a meal.

Paddon-Jones and colleagues (2004) studied the effect of whole protein on muscle protein synthesis. Participants were given a 4-oz beef patty (equivalent to 30 g of protein) and a 12-oz beef patty (about 90 g of protein). In both cases, muscle protein synthesis increased by about 50 percent, suggesting that 30 g of whole protein is an amount at which protein synthesis is already maximized.

Protein Intake Distribution

Data from the 2007–2008 National Health and Nutrition Examination Survey (NHANES) report that adults 70 years and older are consuming an average of 1 g of protein per kilogram of weight per day (ARS, 2010). This amount is broken down to about 20 percent at breakfast, 23 percent at lunch, and 50 percent at dinner. For an average 70-kg person, this equals 14 g of protein at breakfast, 16 g at lunch, and 32 g at dinner. Based on results from the above mentioned controlled studies, this means that on average community-dwelling older adults eat enough protein to stimulate muscle protein synthesis only at dinner. Paddon-Jones and Rasmussen (2009) introduced the theory of an ideal distribution of protein across meals that would maximize protein synthesis and improve muscle protein retention in older adults. Based on findings from previous studies, they proposed that 30 g of protein should be consumed at each of the three major meals. This translates into 1.3 g/kg of protein for a 70-kg person; an amount higher than the Recommended Dietary Allowance (RDA) (0.8 g/kg [IOM, 2002/2005]) and current NHANES data (1.04 g/kg [ARS, 2010]).

Special Considerations for Hospitalized Adults

While healthy older adults tend to lose functionality fairly slowly over time, catastrophic events like falls and illnesses can result in significant losses in muscle mass and physical function. After a catastrophic event, some older adults are unable to return to their initial state of functionality and instead decline toward a state of physical dependence. Hospitalization, as a result of a catastrophic event, causes previously independent older adults to become sedentary, experiencing reductions in number of steps per day and minutes of daily activity. Adults who leave the hospital and increase their steps per day by tenfold are still categorized as sedentary (Fisher et al., 2011).

Longer hospital stays for older adults result in fewer steps per day and more muscle lost. Studies in healthy older adults have shown that 10 days of bed rest induce more muscle loss than 28 days of bed rest in younger adults (9 percent compared to 2 percent) (Kortebein et al., 2007). This muscle mass loss occurred even when the subjects were consuming the RDA for protein of 0.8 g/kg/day. However, older adults in the hospital are not likely to eat an adequate amount of protein to stimulate protein synthesis. Preliminary data (unpublished) from Paddon-Jones' group suggests that older adults in a geriatric hospital that were given a meal containing 40 g of protein only ate about 10 g. On the other hand, a study has shown that protein synthesis can be maintained in older adults through a 10-day bed-rest period when diet is supplemented with 15 g of essential amino acids in addition to the protein RDA (Ferrando et al., 2010).

Closing Remarks

Inadequate protein intake is a predictor of sarcopenia, frailty, and disability. Research shows that muscle protein synthesis in older adults can be stimulated by exercise or intake of about 30 g of protein at each major meal. Additional protein intake above the current RDA may help prevent muscle loss and loss of function in hospitalized older adults. However, further research is needed to determine if the current protein recommendations are adequate to maintain functionality in active, inactive, and hospitalized older adults.

EAT BETTER, MOVE MORE: A COMMUNITY-BASED PROGRAM TO IMPROVE HEALTH BEHAVIORS AMONG OLDER AMERICANS

Presenter: Neva Kirk-Sanchez

The Eat Better, Move More program was a community-based physical activity and nutrition program that was part of the AoA You Can! Steps to Healthier Aging national campaign. The purpose of this program was to encourage older adults participating in community-based programs through the Older Americans Act (OAA) nutrition programs to "take simple steps for better health." National data were collected in order to monitor outcomes among the diverse program population. Neva Kirk-Sanchez, associate professor of clinical physical therapy at the University of Miami Miller School of Medicine, described the development, format, and results of the program as it was implemented by Florida International University in 2005–2006.

Program Format and Development

The program consisted of 12 weekly sessions composed of mini lessons, participatory activities, goal setting, take-home assignments, and incentives. The sessions were designed to encourage people visiting congregate meal sites to participate in a nutrition and physical activity program and improve their health behaviors, such as

- increasing intake of fruits and vegetables,
- increasing calcium and fiber intake,
- eating sensible portion sizes,
- following the food guide pyramid recommendations,
- using pedometers, and
- setting weekly goals to increase the number of daily steps by 10 percent each week in attempts to reach the overall goal of 10,000 steps per week.

Before the national campaign was implemented, two pilot programs tested some aspects of the program. The first pilot program found that older adults would wear pedometers; 80 percent of adults ages 61–90 years with multiple impairments wore them. The second pilot compared the change in daily step count of two groups, one that received pedometers and another that received a preliminary guidebook and educational activities in addition to the pedometers. While both groups increased their number of steps, the latter group showed a larger increase.

Recruitment was targeted to OAA nutrition program sites and elicited through announcements posted on aging websites, distributed through Aging Network listservs, and disseminated through state and local agencies on aging. Of the 106 programs that applied, 10 were chosen to receive the $10,000 grants. Grantees were selected based on size, lack of existing physical activity programs, geographic location, and capacity to collect and report data. A facilitator from each site was trained on protocol implementation and outcome measurement, with a focus on physical activity outcomes since most facilitators were nutritionists. Facilitators discussed successes, challenges, and solutions during biweekly conference calls and through a listserv.

Data Collection and Results

Data were collected on demographics, health conditions, nutrition and physical activity, and activities of daily living (ADLs). In addition, participants completed a Timed Up and Go test (Podsiadlo and Richardson, 1991) and a Health Behavior stages of change questionnaire related to nutrition and physical activity. Of the 999 participants who started the project, 620

(62 percent) completed either the nutrition or the physical activity component (completion rates varied by site from 35 to 85 percent). All of the participants were 60 years or older, except for the Native American participants who were 50 years and older. Fifty-seven percent were Caucasian, 81 percent were women, and the average age was about 74 years (Wellman et al., 2007). The prevalence of chronic conditions was similar to that found in the NHANES except that participants exhibited higher rates of diabetes (19 percent) and arthritis (39 percent), and 53 percent had high or moderate nutrition risk scores. Select data on physical activity participation and limitations in function and activity are as follows:

- 58 percent reported participating in regular activity at least once a week.
- 56 percent agreed they should be more active.
- 63 percent had access to physical activity programs (45 percent participated in those programs).
- 81 percent had access to places to walk (70 percent walked).
- 91 percent had no difficulty with basic ADLs.
- 83 percent had no difficulty with instrumental ADLs.
- 12 percent had some activity limitations due to having fallen in the last month.
- 12 percent used canes.
- 4 percent used walkers (Wellman et al., 2007).

Results from Program Completers Versus Noncompleters

The demographics of the participants who completed the program were nearly identical to those who began the program: 59 percent Caucasian, 25 percent African American, 82 percent women, and an average age of about 75 years. Kirk-Sanchez said people may have dropped out of the program due to the culture of their particular group or the performance of their facilitator. Participants were more likely to adhere to the nutrition component of the program than the physical activity (walking) component. There were only modest differences in the presence of chronic conditions between those who did and did not complete the program. The presence of a chronic condition did not seem to be related to completion of the program, with the exception of much higher rates of reported dizziness among those who dropped out of the physical activity component. She noted that dizziness may be a factor that prevents people from grocery shopping and scanning the shelves. People who dropped out of the program were more likely to

- have difficulty with one or more basic or instrumental ADL,
- be a minority,

- live at or near the poverty level,
- be at nutritional risk,
- have a fear of falling, and
- have lower activity levels, including baseline steps and blocks walked per week.

As compared to those who dropped out of the program, the completers were more likely to be independent in their basic and instrumental ADLs, to have a safe place to walk, and to have incomes above the poverty level. They also had lower nutrition risk scores, reported less fear of falls, and walked more blocks per week and more steps per day at baseline (Wellman et al., 2007). In order to prevent the more frail people from dropping out, Kirk-Sanchez asked, "what kinds of things can we complement the program with? Can they benefit if [they are given] a little extra guidance in either nutrition or physical therapy [or] physical activity?"

Nutrition and Physical Activity Outcomes

Participants who completed the nutrition component of the program increased their intake of fruits, vegetables, calcium-rich foods, fiber-rich foods, and water (see Figure 5-3).

Participants who completed the physical activity component of the program reported increasing the number of blocks walked daily from 10 to 15, the number of stairs climbed daily, their amount of vigorous activity, and their amount of moderate weekend activity. On average, their number of daily steps increased from 3,110 to 4,190—a total of about half a mile per day and a 35 percent increase from week 2 to week 11. Self-reported information was consistent with information obtained from participants' pedometers. On average, participants reported an 8 percent increase in the number of days walked per week from 5.7 at week 2 to 6.2 at week 11. Kirk-Sanchez pointed out that the changes in daily steps were generally made within the first week and sustained throughout the duration of the program.

The Timed Up and Go test consists of a person standing up from sitting in a chair, walking 10 feet, turning around, coming back to the chair, and sitting down. Results from this test are associated with fall risk; if completed in more than 14 seconds, the individual is at a high fall risk (Podsiadlo and Richardson, 1991). The average improvement was significant at 1.38 seconds, which included people who were fairly high functioning at baseline. Among the 113 participants who were in the high fall risk category at baseline, about 39 percent improved to the normal fall risk category with a mean improvement of 3.65 seconds.

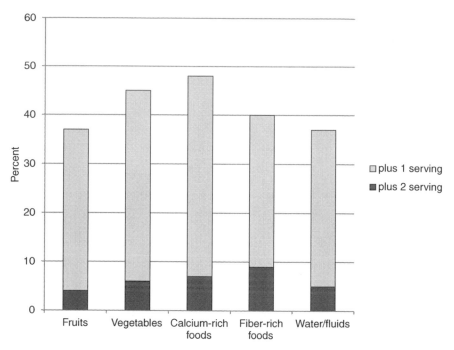

FIGURE 5-3 Percentage of participants that increased their intake of foods and water.
SOURCE: Wellman et al., 2007.

Stages of Change Outcomes

Participants who completed the nutrition component were asked questions related to their readiness to change their intake of calcium-rich foods. More than half (56 percent) increased one or more stages, including 61 percent who moved from the Preparation to the Action or Maintenance stage. There was a threefold increase in the number of people in the Action stage and a 6 percent increase in the Maintenance stage.

Similar changes were seen among those who completed the physical activity component; 67 percent increased by one more stage and 35 percent increased by more than two stages. Three-quarters of participants moved from the Preparation stage to the Action or Maintenance stage, and the number of people in the Pre-Contemplation and Contemplation stages decreased by 21 percent. "This is great news. We really changed people's attitudes. We seemed to change people's behavior. Changes were modest in some cases, but I think it's important to note that," said Kirk-Sanchez.

Follow-Up to Eat Better, Move More

In response to requests for more weekly modules, a second part of Eat Better, Move More was published online and translated into Spanish. It includes updated nutrition information on the 2005 *Dietary Guidelines for Americans* (HHS and USDA, 2005), the DASH diet (NHLBI, 2006), and nutrients of concern, including vitamins D and B_{12} and potassium. Additional physical activity recommendations were added related to stretching, balance, strengthening, use of an exercise band, and continued use of pedometers (Kamp et al., 2007).

Kirk-Sanchez and the group at Florida International University also conducted a small pilot study with 30 older subjects (average age of 82 years), 14 of which completed the 12-week intervention. Results included an average improvement of 2.3 seconds in the Timed Up and Go test, an increase of 83 meters in the timed 6-minute walk, and an increase of 4 repetitions in the timed bicep curls. Due to the small sample size, changes in nutrition behaviors could not be assessed.

Kirk-Sanchez closed by suggesting that future steps include conducting a larger and more controlled pilot study of Eat Better, Move More Part 2 with a focus on special populations, such as Latinos and people with specific chronic conditions, and additional outcomes including depression and cognition.

DISCUSSION

Moderator: Douglas Paddon-Jones

During the discussion, points raised by participants included protein intake and recommendations, and aspects of MNT.

Chronic Versus Acute Feeding of Protein

Robert Russell revisited the idea of changing the Dietary Reference Intakes (DRIs) for protein and asked, since changes in Estimated Average Requirements are based on chronic feeding experiments, if there were data on chronic feeding of protein over the 33 percent distribution that was presented. Volpi responded that those data do not currently exist and agreed that more studies in that area need to be conducted. Paddon-Jones agreed and added that he has nearly completed a study comparing 24-hour protein synthesis among people on an evenly distributed diet to those on a skewed "carbohydrate breakfast diet." He said they hope to tie those results to nitrogen balance in order to reevaluate the protein DRIs. Volpi noted that the distribution of protein intake in nitrogen balance studies is highly controlled and evenly distributed, unlike the pattern of protein intake in peoples' diets. Studies, such as NHANES, should not focus on total daily intake since it obscures variability throughout the day; rather they should look at distribution of intake, she suggested.

Volpi noted that animal proteins are higher quality than plant proteins because they contain a proportion of amino acids, particularly essential amino acids, that is similar to that of our bodies. There have been small acute studies and short-term clinical trials that compared proteins and how protein quality is measured. For example, dairy protein is slightly better at stimulating protein synthesis than soy protein, and lower-quality proteins, such as wheat and chickpea, are less digestible. She suggested that the type of protein be considered when measuring intake and making recommendations.

Revisions to the *Dietary Guidelines for Americans'* Recommendations for Protein Intake by Older Adults

Adele Hite observed that several presenters suggested that the DRI recommendation for protein intake for older adults may not be appropriate. She expressed concern since the DRIs are the basis for federal nutrition policy, programs, and research. Volpi said that more studies need to be conducted that vigorously test different protein intake distribution patterns among older adults.

Therapeutic Meals

Robert Miller asked Troyer to elaborate on a description of the therapeutic meals and whether people without hypertension received low-sodium or low-fat meals. Troyer said that all participants received low-sodium DASH diet meals designed for people with hypertension. Miller commented that palatability may be an issue for people who did not require low-sodium meals. Troyer said that they conducted some follow-up with regard to what the participants were eating; however, they do not know if recipients added anything to the meals, such as butter or salt.

Cost Effectiveness of MNT

Mary Pat Raimondi commented that, based on her work on the reauthorization of the OAA, cost data related to return on investment are needed by legislators. She was directed to data presented in two articles in the *Journal of the American Dietetic Association*, by Troyer (Troyer et al., 2010b) and Nancy Cohen (Delahanty et al., 2001). Cost-effectiveness values are based on quantity and quality of life gained and include dimensions of health such as mobility, depression, and social functioning.

REFERENCES

Appel, L. J., T. J. Moore, E. Obarzanek, W. M. Vollmer, L. P. Svetkey, F. M. Sacks, G. A. Bray, T. M. Vogt, J. A. Cutler, M. M. Windhauser, P. H. Lin, N. Karanja, D. Simons-Morton, M, McCullough, I, Swain, P. Steele, M. A. Evans, E. R. Miller III, and B. W. Harsha. 1997. A clinical trial of the effects of dietary patterns on blood pressure. *New England Journal of Medicine* 336(16):1117–1124.

ARS (Agricultural Research Service). 2010. *What We Eat in America, NHANES 2007-2008: Table 5.* Washington, DC. http://www.ars.usda.gov/SP2UserFiles/Place/12355000/pdf/0708/Table_5_EIN_GEN_07.pdf (accessed December 12, 2011).

Bandura, A. 1986. *Social Foundations of Thought and Action: A Social Cognitive Theory.* Englewood Cliffs, NJ: Prentice Hall.

Baron, M. 2005. Reducing drug usage and adverse effects: Part III: Cardiovascular disease and hyperlipidemia. *Health Care Food & Nutrition* 22(6):7–11.

Blumenthal, J. A., M. A. Babyak, A. Hinderliter, L. L. Watkins, L. Craighead, P. H. Lin, C. Caccia, J. Johnson, R. Waugh, and A. Sherwood. 2010. Effects of the DASH diet alone and in combination with exercise and weight loss on blood pressure and cardiovascular biomarkers in men and women with high blood pressure: The ENCORE study. *Archives of Internal Medicine* 170(2):126–135.

Braithwaite, R. S., D. O. Meltzer, J. T. King, D. Leslie, and M. S. Roberts. 2008. What does the value of modern medicine say about the $50,000 per quality-adjusted life-year decision rule? *Medical Care* 46(4):349–356.

Brown, J. S., R. Wing, E. Barrett-Connor, L. M. Nyberg, J. W. Kusek, T. J. Orchard, Y. Ma, E. Vittinghoff, and A. M. Kanaya. 2006. Lifestyle intervention is associated with lower prevalence of urinary incontinence: The Diabetes Prevention Program. *Diabetes Care* 29(2):385–390.

Crandall, J., D. Schade, Y. Ma, W. Y. Fujimoto, E. Barrett-Connor, S. Fowler, S. Dagogo-Jack, and R. Andres. 2006. The influence of age on the effects of lifestyle modification and metformin in prevention of diabetes. *Journal of Gerontology—Series A Biological Sciences and Medical Sciences* 61(10):1075–1081.

Delahanty, L. M., I. M. Sonnenberg, D. Hayden, and D. M. Nathan. 2001. Clinical and cost outcomes of medical nutrition therapy for hypercholesterolemia: A controlled trial. *Journal of the American Dietetic Association* 101(9):1012–1023.

Delahanty, L. M., D. Hayden, A. Ammerman, and D. M. Nathan. 2002. Medical nutrition therapy for hypercholesterolemia positively affects patient satisfaction and quality of life outcomes. *Annals of Behavioral Medicine* 24(4):269–278.

Diabetes Prevention Program Research Group. 2009. 10-year follow-up of diabetes incidence and weight loss in the Diabetes Prevention Program Outcomes Study. *The Lancet* 374(9702):1677–1686.

Dickinson, H. O., J. M. Mason, D. J. Nicolson, F. Campbell, F. R. Beyer, J. V. Cook, B. Williams, and G. A. Ford. 2006. Lifestyle interventions to reduce raised blood pressure: A systematic review of randomized controlled trials. *Journal of Hypertension* 24(2):215–223.

Elmer, P. J., E. Obarzanek, W. M. Vollmer, D. Simons-Morton, V. J. Stevens, D. R. Young, P. H. Lin, C. Champagne, D. W. Harsha, L. P. Svetkey, J. Ard, P. J. Brantley, M. A. Proschan, T. P. Erlinger, and L. J. Appel. 2006. Effects of comprehensive lifestyle modification on diet, weight, physical fitness, and blood pressure control: 18-month results of a randomized trial. *Annals of Internal Medicine* 144(7):485–495.

Ferrando, A. A., D. Paddon-Jones, N. P. Hays, P. Kortebein, O. Ronsen, R. H. Williams, A. McComb, T. B. Symons, R. R. Wolfe, and W. Evans. 2010. EAA supplementation to increase nitrogen intake improves muscle function during bed rest in the elderly. *Clinical Nutrition* 29(1):18–23.

Fisher, E. B., E. A. Walker, A. Bostrom, B. Fischhoff, D. Haire-Joshu, and S. B. Johnson. 2002. Behavioral science research in the prevention of diabetes: Status and opportunities. *Diabetes Care* 25(3):599–606.

Fisher, S. R., J. S. Goodwin, E. J. Protas, Y. F. Kuo, J. E. Graham, K. J. Ottenbacher, and G. V. Ostir. 2011. Ambulatory activity of older adults hospitalized with acute medical illness. *Journal of the American Geriatrics Society* 59(1):91–95.

Franz, M. J., J. L. Boucher, J. Green-Pastors, and M. A. Powers. 2008. Evidence-based nutrition practice guidelines for diabetes and scope and standards of practice. *Journal of the American Dietetic Association* 108(4 Suppl.):S52–S58.

Fujita, S., E. L. Glynn, K. L. Timmerman, B. B. Rasmussen, and E. Volpi. 2009. Supraphysiological hyperinsulinaemia is necessary to stimulate skeletal muscle protein anabolism in older adults: Evidence of a true age-related insulin resistance of muscle protein metabolism. *Diabetologia* 52(9):1889–1898.

Gehling, E. 2001. Medical nutrition therapy: An individualized approach to treating diabetes. *Lippincott's Case Management: Managing the Process of Patient Care* 6(1):2–9; quiz 10–12.

HHS and USDA (U.S. Department of Health and Human Services and U.S. Department of Agriculture). 2005. Dietary Guidelines for Americans. Washington, DC: U.S. Government Printing Office. http://www.health.gov/DietaryGuidelines/dga2005/document/ (accessed November 21, 2011).

Houston, D. K., B. J. Nicklas, J. Ding, T. B. Harris, F. A. Tylavsky, A. B. Newman, S. L. Jung, N. R. Sahyoun, M. Visser, and S. B. Kritchevsky. 2008. Dietary protein intake is associated with lean mass change in older, community-dwelling adults: The Health, Aging, and Body Composition (Health ABC) study. *American Journal of Clinical Nutrition* 87(1):150–155.

IOM (Institute of Medicine). 2000. *The Role of Nutrition in Maintaining Health in the Nation's Elderly: Evaluating Coverage of Nutrition Services for the Medicare Population.* Washington, DC: National Academy Press.

IOM. 2002/2005. *Dietary Reference Intakes for Energy, Carbohydrate, Fiber, Fat, Fatty Acids, Cholesterol, Protein, and Amino Acids.* Washington, DC: The National Academies Press.

Kamp, B., N. Kirk-Sanchez, S. Dukes, and N. Wellman. 2007. *Eat Better, Move More: Part 2.* Miami, FL: Florida International University. http://nutritionandaging.fiu.edu/You_Can/YouCanGuide_PART_2.pdf (accessed December 12, 2011).

Katsanos, C. S., H. Kobayashi, M. Sheffield-Moore, A. Aarsland, and R. R. Wolfe. 2006. A high proportion of leucine is required for optimal stimulation of the rate of muscle protein synthesis by essential amino acids in the elderly. *American Journal of Physiology-Endocrinology and Metabolism* 291(2):E381–E387.

Knowler, W. C., E. Barrett-Connor, S. E. Fowler, R. F. Hamman, J. M. Lachin, E. A. Walker, and D. M. Nathan. 2002. Reduction in the incidence of type 2 diabetes with lifestyle intervention or metformin. *New England Journal of Medicine* 346(5):393–403.

Kortebein, P., A. Ferrando, J. Lombeida, R. Wolfe, and W. J. Evans. 2007. Effect of 10 days of bed rest on skeletal muscle in healthy older adults. *Journal of the American Medical Association* 297(16):1772–1774.

Lim, H. J., Y. M. Choi, and R. Choue. 2008. Dietary intervention with emphasis on folate intake reduces serum lipids but not plasma homocysteine levels in hyperlipidemic patients. *Nutrition Research* 28(11):767–774.

Lin, P. H., L. J. Appel, K. Funk, S. Craddick, C. Chen, P. Elmer, M. A. McBurnie, and C. Champagne. 2007. The PREMIER intervention helps participants follow the Dietary Approaches to Stop Hypertension dietary pattern and the current Dietary Reference Intakes recommendations. *Journal of the American Dietetic Association* 107(9):1541–1551.

McCaffree, J. 2003. Position of the American Dietetic Association: Integration of medical nutrition therapy and pharmacotherapy. *Journal of the American Dietetic Association* 103(10):1363–1370.

Michael, P. 2001. Impact and components of the Medicare MNT benefit. *Journal of the American Dietetic Association* 101(10):1140–1141.

Newman, A. B., V. Kupelian, M. Visser, E. M. Simonsick, B. H. Goodpaster, S. B. Kritchevsky, F. A. Tylavsky, S. M. Rubin, and T. B. Harris. 2006. Strength, but not muscle mass, is associated with mortality in the Health, Aging and Body Composition study cohort. *Journal of Gerontology— Series A, Biological Sciences and Medical Sciences* 61(1):72–77.

NHLBI (National Heart, Lung, and Blood Institute). 2006. *Your Guide to Lowering Your Blood Pressure with DASH.* http://www.nhlbi.nih.gov/health/public/heart/hbp/dash/new_dash.pdf (accessed November 21, 2011).

Paddon-Jones, D., and B. B. Rasmussen. 2009. Dietary protein recommendations and the prevention of sarcopenia. *Current Opinion in Clinical Nutrition and Metabolic Care* 12(1):86–90.

Paddon-Jones, D., M. Sheffield-Moore, X. J. Zhang, E. Volpi, S. E. Wolf, A. Aarsland, A. A. Ferrando, and R. R. Wolfe. 2004. Amino acid ingestion improves muscle protein synthesis in the young and elderly. *American Journal of Physiology-Endocrinology and Metabolism* 286(3):E321–E328.

Pavlovich, W. D., H. Waters, W. Weller, and E. B. Bass. 2004. Systematic review of literature on the cost-effectiveness of nutrition services. *Journal of the American Dietetic Association* 104(2):226–232.

Peyrot, M., and R. R. Rubin. 2007. Behavioral and psychosocial interventions in diabetes: A conceptual review. *Diabetes Care* 30(10):2433–2440.

Podsiadlo, D., and S. Richardson. 1991. The timed "Up and Go": A test of basic functional mobility for frail elderly persons. *Journal of the American Geriatrics Society* 39(2):142–148.

Racine, E., J. L. Troyer, J. Warren-Findlow, and W. J. McAuley. 2011. The effect of medical nutrition therapy on changes in dietary knowledge and DASH diet adherence in older adults with cardiovascular disease. *Journal of Nutrition, Health and Aging* 15(10):1–9.

Rasmussen, B. B., S. Fujita, R. R. Wolfe, B. Mittendorfer, M. Roy, V. L. Rowe, and E. Volpi. 2006. Insulin resistance of muscle protein metabolism in aging. *FASEB Journal* 20(6):768–769.

Rezabek, K. M. 2001. Medical nutrition therapy in type 2 diabetes. *Nursing Clinics of North America* 36(2):203–216, vi.

Roubenoff, R., and C. Castaneda. 2001. Sarcopenia—Understanding the dynamics of aging muscle. *Journal of the American Medical Association* 286(10):1230–1231.

Sacks, F. M., L. P. Svetkey, W. M. Vollmer, L. J. Appel, G. A. Bray, D. Harsha, E. Obarzanek, P. R. Conlin, E. R. Miller III, D. G. Simons-Morton, N. Karanja, P. H. Lin, M. Aickin, M. M. Most-Windhauser, T. J. Moore, M. A. Proschan, and J. A. Cutler. 2001. Effects on blood pressure of reduced dietary sodium and the Dietary Approaches to Stop Hypertension (DASH) diet. *New England Journal of Medicine* 344(1):3–10.

Schechter, C. B., C. E. Basch, A. Caban, and E. A. Walker. 2008. Cost effectiveness of a telephone intervention to promote dilated fundus examination in adults with diabetes mellitus. *Clinical Ophthalmology* 2(4):763–768.

Sikand, G., M. L. Kashyap, N. D. Wong, and J. C. Hsu. 2000. Dietitian intervention improves lipid values and saves medication costs in men with combined hyperlipidemia and a history of niacin noncompliance. *Journal of the American Dietetic Association* 100(2):218–224.

Stokols, D. 1996. Translating social ecological theory into guidelines for community health promotion. *American Journal of Health Promotion* 10(4):282–298.

Timmerman, K. L., J. L. Lee, H. C. Dreyer, S. Dhanani, E. L. Glynn, C. S. Fry, M. J. Drummond, M. Sheffield-Moore, B. B. Rasmussen, and E. Volpi. 2010a. Insulin stimulates human skeletal muscle protein synthesis via an indirect mechanism involving endothelial-dependent vasodilation and mammalian target of rapamycin complex 1 signaling. *Journal of Clinical Endocrinology and Metabolism* 95(8):3848–3857.

Timmerman, K. L., J. L. Lee, S. Fujita, S. Dhanani, H. C. Dreyer, C. S. Fry, M. J. Drummond, M. Sheffield-Moore, B. B. Rasmussen, and E. Volpi. 2010b. Pharmacological vasodilation improves insulin-stimulated muscle protein anabolism but not glucose utilization in older adults. *Diabetes* 59(11):2764–2771.

Toobert, D. J., and R. E. Glasgow. 1994. Assessing diabetes self-management: The summary of diabetes self-care activities questionnaire. In *Handbook of Psychology and Diabetes*, edited by C. Bradley. Chur, Switzerland: Hardood Academic.

Troyer, J. L. 2011. Nutrition intervention for cardiovascular disease: Home-delivered medical nutrition therapy and DASH. Presented at the Institute of Medicine Workshop on Nutrition and Healthy Aging in the Community. Washington, DC, October 5–6.

Troyer, J. L., E. F. Racine, G. W. Ngugi, and W. J. McAuley. 2010a. The effect of home-delivered Dietary Approach to Stop Hypertension (DASH) meals on the diets of older adults with cardiovascular disease. *American Journal of Clinical Nutrition* 91(5):1204–1212.

Troyer, J. L., W. J. McAuley, and M. E. McCutcheon. 2010b. Cost-effectiveness of medical nutrition therapy and therapeutically designed meals for older adults with cardiovascular disease. *Journal of the American Dietetic Association* 110(12):1840–1851.

Volpi, E., B. Mittendorfer, B. B. Rasmussen, and R. R. Wolfe. 2000. The response of muscle protein anabolism to combined hyperaminoacidemia and glucose-induced hyperinsulinemia is impaired in the elderly. *Journal of Clinical Endocrinology and Metabolism* 85(12):4481–4490.

Wagner, E. H. 1998. Chronic disease management: What will it take to improve care for chronic illness? *Effective Clinical Practice* 1(1):2–4.

Wagner, E. H., B. T. Austin, C. Davis, M. Hindmarsh, J. Schaefer, and A. Bonomi. 2001. Improving chronic illness care: Translating evidence into action. *Health Affairs* 20(6):64–78.

Walker, F. A., C. B. Schechter, A. Caban, and C. E. Basch. 2008. Telephone intervention to promote diabetic retinopathy screening among the urban poor. *American Journal of Preventive Medicine* 34(3):185–191.

Walker, E. A., C. Shmukler, R. Ullman, E. Blanco, M. Scollan-Koliopoulus, and H. W. Cohen. 2011. Results of a successful telephonic intervention to improve diabetes control in urban adults: A randomized trial. *Diabetes Care* 34(1):2–7.

Wellman, N. S., B. Kamp, N. J. Kirk-Sanchez, and P. M. Johnson. 2007. Eat Better & Move More: A community-based program designed to improve diets and increase physical activity among older Americans. *American Journal of Public Health* 97(4):710–717.

Wing, R. R. 2004. Achieving weight and activity goals among Diabetes Prevention Program lifestyle participants. *Obesity Research* 12(9):1426–1434.

Wylie-Rosett, J., and L. Delahanty. 2002. An integral role of the dietitian: Implications of the Diabetes Prevention Program. *Journal of the American Dietetic Association* 102(8):1065–1068.

6

Research Gaps

The final session consisted of a panel discussion addressing research gaps in knowledge about nutrition interventions and services for older adults in the community setting. The discussion was moderated by Nancy S. Wellman, from Tufts University, and included presentations by panel members Mary Ann Johnson from the University of Georgia, Rebecca Costello from the National Institutes of Health (NIH) Office of Dietary Supplements (ODS), Robert M. Russell from the NIH ODS and Tufts University, and Judy Hannah from the NIH National Institute on Aging (NIA). Each panel member had been asked to identify what they perceived to be the top three areas in which research is needed on nutrition issues and aging. Their presentations were followed by an open discussion period. The research gaps identified during this session are summarized below.

EDUCATION OF DIETITIANS

Mary Ann Johnson opened the panel discussion by addressing the need for educating future dietitians on issues related to aging. While the registered dietitian is the expert in food and nutrition services and interventions, nutrition is only one of the many issues that a client or patient will experience. She called for broad training and exposure to the many problems older people face. She also stressed that dietitians need an appreciation of related social and health professions so they can function effectively within health care teams and systems that serve older adults. Wellman agreed that more should be done to educate future dietitians about aging, noting that other health professions have multiple undergraduate and graduate courses on aging.

NUTRITION SERVICES FOR OLDER ADULTS

Johnson also called for the integration of food and nutrition care and services among all settings, including community, outpatient, rehabilitation, assisted living, and nursing homes. Older adults who need nutrition services should be targeted through well-designed screening programs. Interventions need to be developed and implemented that are tailored to diverse cultures, geographic locations, and characteristics of older adults in those settings. Johnson believes patient-directed services, with a dietitian or health care provider functioning as a coach, will likely be embraced by older adults. Elizabeth Walker suggested research on how to educate people to make competent health-related decisions, such as selecting nutrition services as a patient-directed benefit.

Judy Simon raised the issue of the disconnect between the requirement that meals provided by the Older Americans Act (OAA) Nutrition Program meet current dietary guidelines and the food preferences of older adults. She suggested research examine how to bridge that gap and determine if different meal standards and more palatable meals would attract more people into the declining congregate meal programs. She added that it is essential to determine the effect of changing dietary guidelines on program costs. Very few caterers bid on providing foods for these programs because it is not cost-effective to prepare these meals since the nutrition programs are small and have restrictions related to nutrient requirements.

REFINING OUTCOME MEASURES

Another research gap identified by Johnson is the refinement of outcome measures for interventions to demonstrate cost effectiveness and improved quality of life. Robert Russell concurred and, as noted earlier in the workshop, pointed out that one of the major goals of the Administration on Aging (AoA) is to have people remain in their homes as long as possible instead of going into a nursing home. However, the evaluations of AoA programs have been small in scale and have not addressed the main interest of Congress—do the interventions prevent people from being institutionalized and reduce health care expenses? Furthermore, if current evaluations tying these programs to Medicare and Medicaid outcomes show ineffectiveness and do not result in reduced health care spending, it must be determined why they are unsuccessful so improvements can be made.

Wellman also emphasized the need for more outcome data on the cost effectiveness of the OAA Nutrition Program. About 40 percent of older adults who participate in the home-delivered meal program are in and out of the hospital during the year. She proposed that many of these homebound people should be identified through nutrition assessment at the hospital and provided more than just five lunches a week. It is necessary to document Medicare and Medicaid cost savings for those whose food and other service needs are met through the program. The importance of documenting outcomes should be made clear to the local staff who carry out the OAA Nutrition Program.

Wellman compared the OAA program to the Special Supplemental Nutrition Program for Women, Infants, and Children (WIC). Both federal programs started in the 1970s. Federal funding for WIC has increased 332-fold, Wellman reported, while funding for OAA has increased only sixfold. She attributed this difference partially to the fact that evaluations of the WIC program demonstrated cost savings from the beginning. Early data revealed that for every dollar spent in WIC, $3 were saved in intensive care unit dollars. Nadine Sahyoun noted that the WIC program is an established national program and the participants are not sick, making it somewhat easier to follow and have an end point. Alternatively, the OAA Nutrition Program is a grassroots program and many participants have chronic conditions and may be frail. The aging network is complicated because programs vary by state and locales; therefore, innovations may be required to determine what outcomes to measure.

Judy Hannah noted that government recognizes that most of a person's health care expenditures occur in the last 2 years of his or her lifespan. Therefore, she stressed that the focus of programs and research must be to ensure health related quality of life, to keep people in their homes instead of institutions, and to reduce health care costs.

USE OF FORTIFIED FOODS AND DIETARY SUPPLEMENTS

Johnson pointed to the need to conduct basic and translational research on the development, evaluation, and appropriate use of fortified foods and dietary supplements to maintain and enhance health and well-being. She said there is a need to establish an evidence base for specific nutrients and supplements with an evidence base of effectiveness and to help health care professionals and consumers make appropriate choices. Rebecca Costello suggested the creation of informational databases on dietary supplements for this same reason. She also acknowledged the continued need for development of relational databases that address structural-activity relationships and are populated with biochemical, toxicological, and dietary supplement information.

Costello reported that data from the 2003–2006 National Health and Nutrition Examination Survey (NHANES) cycle revealed that 54 percent of adults consume dietary supplements, with 70 percent of adults over 71 years of age using them. She presented on the progress made related to the research gaps identified at a 2003 NIH conference on dietary supplements in older adults. The first was further characterization of dietary supplement usage behaviors, including the need to describe the effect of caregivers' advice. While some newer data have been reported, the need still exists to collect data on caregivers. There is also a need to characterize the diversity of beliefs (e.g., alternative medicine) and behavioral, cultural, and social factors that can affect and confound dietary supplement data. Costello identified various entities (or groups) that have collected this type of data, including the Centers for Disease Control and Prevention's 2002 National Health Interview Survey and NHANES, the Jackson Heart Study, the Women's Health Initiative, and the Gingko Evaluation of Memory Study. Nevertheless, there is an ongoing need to evaluate dietary supplement use as well as the methods for the collection of dietary supplement data.

Another research gap that remains, according to Costello, includes preclinical and clinical studies to

- better distinguish which population groups of older adults may need dietary supplements,
- evaluate supplement safety and efficacy,
- capture usual dietary intakes and total daily intakes of nutrients,
- evaluate drug-nutrient interactions, and
- determine micronutrient needs of an aging population.

NUTRIENT REQUIREMENTS

Costello identified another research gap as the need for improved methodologies, including biomarkers, analytical methods, diet assessment tools, and systematic reviews. While progress has been made on the validation of biologic markers used in national surveys, such as the NHANES collection of data on biochemistry for folic acid and vitamin D assessments, similar work must be done for other nutrients that may be of public health importance for older adults. Costello reported significant developments in the area of analytic methods. The ODS Analytical Methods and Reference Materials Program has supported the development and validation of reference standards for a host of dietary supplements and supplement constituents. In particular, the program collaborated on the development and use of a National Institute of Standards and Technology Vitamin D standard. Costello noted that it is still necessary to determine the best way to incorporate formal methods of weighing the evidence for interpretation into policy and clinical practice. Multiple groups, such as the Agency for Healthcare Quality and Research, NIH, the U.S. Department of Agriculture (USDA), the American Dietetic Association, and most recently the Institute of Medicine (IOM), have explored the methodology for evaluating, tabulating, and interpreting the evidence base for dietary supplements.

Russell identified research on nutrient requirements as a priority research gap, explaining that some current Dietary Reference Intakes (DRIs) are "clearly wrong." For example, the Estimated Average Requirements (EARs) for vitamin E (and probably vitamin A) are too high; continued research and improved biomarkers are needed to obtain more realistic and accurate EARs. Additionally, evidence suggests that the Recommended Dietary Allowance (RDA) for vitamin B_{12} might be too low; European trials indicate that older adults may need as much as 6 µg per day. As mentioned earlier in the workshop, vitamin D has been linked to diseases other than bone disease. However, after an exhaustive review of the evidence the IOM Committee to Review DRIs for Vitamin D and Calcium found that the evidence supported a role for these nutrients in bone health but not in other conditions. Macronutrient requirements must also be studied further, as highlighted by the discussion of protein requirements during the workshop (see Chapter 5).

Russell pointed out that safe upper levels of nutrients must also be evaluated in light of the elevated usage of dietary supplements by older adults; for example, as mentioned by Katherine Tucker, folate intake is a concern (see Chapter 2). Furthermore, as more products are developed with nanotechnology, the bioavailability of certain nutrients will be enhanced and adjustments in RDAs or EARs may be needed to compensate for increased bioavailability.

NUTRITION AND COGNITION

Russell identified nutrition and cognition as a research priority that should continue to be addressed. Current research focuses mainly on the B vitamins, particularly vitamin B_{12} and folate; however, increasing the thiamine requirement should be considered because many older people use diuretics, which increase the loss of thiamine in the urine. Furthermore, he explained that there are recent data showing some B vitamins can slow the progression of early dementia and brain atrophy in individuals with high homocysteine levels. Russell stated that further research should be conducted on the relationship between cognition and the B vitamins, omega-3 fatty acids, and vitamin D, and that good biomarkers need to be developed.

COMMUNICATION AND EDUCATION

According to a workshop participant, another area for development is communication with caregivers and educational materials that are amenable to older adults' needs as nutrition science evolves. For example, information on how USDA's "MyPlate" (http://www.choosemyplate.gov) translates to the older American diet would be helpful. Additionally, there is a need to effectively communicate best practice approaches to implementation of these recommendations for the patient and the patient's family. Messages can be very confusing as patients move through the health care system continuum from community to hospital(s), therefore, the use of common language would be helpful.

Sahyoun said that more outreach to the most vulnerable people in the aging population is necessary. Referring to James Hester's discussion on the three silos in the transition of care (see Chapter 4), she commented that in times of recession it would be beneficial to use available linkages and resources to increase awareness of existing programs and services. However, since funding is limited, a method of prioritization to serve the people most in need of assistance would have to be established.

OBESITY AND RELATED DISORDERS

Prevention and treatment of obesity and obesity-related disorders (including sarcopenic obesity) across the spectrum of health and functional status was another area of research identified by Johnson and Russell. Johnson noted that the increase in the aging population is colliding with the epidemic of obesity and suggested that failure to address the problem of obesity in older adults may even erode some of the gains made in life expectancy in the past century.

FOOD INSECURITY AND HEALTHY AGING

Referring to James Ziliak's presentation on *Food Insecurity Among Older Americans*, Johnson emphasized that the basic food needs of older adults must be met, noting that nutrition interventions cannot work if people cannot access, afford, or prepare the foods they need. Connie Bales, questioning the current recession's impact on food insecurity in older adults, worried that they may be overlooked in light of concerns for children and suggested the examination of ways to prioritize the needs of many. Nancy Cohen stated that the study of food deserts is important, with focus on policy changes that communities can make to enhance food availability and food access. Karen Jackson Holzhauer identified the role of community gardens, local produce, and food banks in increasing food availability in food deserts. Sustainability of such programs and their impact on the quality of life and food would need to be measured. A related issue to be examined, according to Elizabeth Walker, is "food swamps," urban areas with a large concentration of fast food outlets.

FUNDING OPPORTUNITY

Judy Hannah concluded the presentations by providing information on an NIA/AoA funding announcement for R01 applications. The topic of research for this funding is *Translational Research to Help Older Adults Maintain Their Health and Independence in the Community*. Hannah noted that the goal of this funding is to move the evaluation of well-documented, evidence-based interventions from a strict research setting into community settings, thus forming a true partnership. Two of the requirements listed in the announcement are (1) a link between the university and organizations working with older adults in the community and (2) cost effectiveness as one of the criteria. Nutrition is one of a variety of criteria that can be evaluated.

OTHER RESEARCH GAPS

Marketing research is another significant gap identified by workshop participants. Mary Pat Raimondi believes that more focus groups with older adults should be conducted to determine what foods appeal to them and to identify other issues of concern. She also suggested addressing marketing claims since there is a lack of trust by older consumers.

Holzhauer proposed studying how the sensory appreciation of foods by older adults and plate appeal could change the way older adults eat.

Russell mentioned the effect of microbiomes on human metabolism and disease is a relatively new area of research to explore.

Douglas Paddon-Jones provided a different viewpoint on research gaps; quite often knowledge of the interface between practitioners and patients is lacking from a researcher's perspective. Forums such as this workshop provide an opportunity to inform researchers on how to adapt their research to best meet the needs of practitioners and, ultimately, their patients.

A

Workshop Agenda

NUTRITION AND HEALTHY AGING IN THE COMMUNITY WORKSHOP AGENDA

The Holiday Inn Central
Washington, DC
October 5–6, 2011

WORKSHOP PURPOSE

1. Address the strengths and limitations of community-based delivery of nutrition services for older persons
2. Identify beneficial nutrition interventions and model programs
   a. To promote successful transition from acute, subacute, and chronic care to home
   b. To promote health and independent living in the community
3. Highlight needed research priorities

Wednesday, October 5, 2011: Day 1

INTRODUCTION

8:30–8:40 a.m. Welcome, Introductions, and Purpose
Gordon L. Jensen
Workshop Moderator and Planning Committee Chair
Pennsylvania State University

8:40–9:10 The Aging Landscape in the Community Setting
Edwin L. Walker
Administration on Aging

9:10–9:15   The Importance of Nutrition Care in the Community
               Setting: Case Study
               Elizabeth B. Landon
               CareLink

SESSION 1:
NUTRITION ISSUES OF CONCERN IN THE COMMUNITY

9:15–9:20   Introduction by Moderator
               Connie W. Bales
               Duke University
               Durham Veterans Administration Medical Center

9:20–9:40   Nutrition Screening at Discharge and in the Community
               Joseph R. Sharkey
               Texas A&M Health Sciences Center

9:40–10:00   Food Insecurity Among Older Americans
               James P. Ziliak
               University of Kentucky

10:00–10:15   Break

10:15–10:35   Sarcopenic Obesity and Aging
               Gordon L. Jensen
               Pennsylvania State University

10:35–10:55   Dietary Patterns for Aging Adults
               Katherine L. Tucker
               Northeastern University

10:55–11:15   Economic and Resource Issues Surrounding Nutrition
               Services for Older Persons in the Community Setting
               Kathryn Larin
               Government Accountability Office

11:15–11:45   Speaker Panel with Audience Participation

11:45 a.m.– 12:30 p.m.	Nutrition Issues Related to Aging in the Community: Perspectives and Open Discussion Moderator: Gordon L. Jensen
	Robert H. Miller *Abbott Nutrition*
	Jean Lloyd *Administration on Aging*
	Enid A. Borden *Meals On Wheels Association of America* *Meals On Wheels Research Foundation*
12:30–1:45	Lunch

SESSION 2: TRANSITION CARE AND BEYOND

1:45–1:50	Introduction by Moderator Nadine R. Sahyoun *University of Maryland*
1:50–2:10	Role of Nutrition in Hospital Discharge Planning: Current and Potential Contribution of the Dietitian Charlene Compher *University of Pennsylvania*
2:10–2:30	Transition Care: A Multidisciplinary Approach Eric A. Coleman *University of Colorado at Denver*
2:30–2:50	Nutrition in Home- and Community-Based Systems State by State Bobbie L. Morris *Alabama Department of Senior Services*
2:50–3:10	Speaker Panel with Audience Participation
3:10–3:25	Break

SESSION 3: TRANSITION TO COMMUNITY CARE: MODELS AND OPPORTUNITIES

3:25–3:30   **Introduction by Moderator**
                 Julie L. Locher
                 University of Alabama at Birmingham

3:30–3:50   **Innovations in Care Transitions: An Overview**
                 James A. Hester
                 Innovation Center, Centers for Medicare and Medicaid Services

3:50–4:10   **Veterans Directed Home- and Community-Based Services**
                 Daniel J. Schoeps
                 Geriatrics and Extended Care, Veterans Administration Central Office
                 Lori Gerhard
                 Administration on Aging

4:10–4:30   **Transitional Care in Canada**
                 Heather Keller
                 University of Waterloo

4:30–4:50   **Speaker Panel with Audience Participation**

4:50–5:00   **Wrap Up and Adjourn**

Thursday, October 6, 2011: Day 2

SESSION 4: SUCCESSFUL INTERVENTION MODELS IN THE COMMUNITY SETTING

8:30–8:35 a.m.   Introduction by Moderator
                 Douglas Paddon-Jones
                 University of Texas Medical Branch

8:35–8:55   **Diabetes Self-Management Support in the Community: Healthy Eating Considerations**
                 Elizabeth A. Walker
                 Albert Einstein College of Medicine

8:55–9:15	Nutrition Intervention for Cardiovascular Disease Jennifer L. Troyer *University of North Carolina at Charlotte*
9:15–9:35	Nutrition Intervention for Sarcopenia and Frailty Elena Volpi *University of Texas Medical Branch*
9:35–9:55	Eat Better, Move More: A Community-Based Program to Improve Diets and Increase Physical Activity Neva Kirk-Sanchez *University of Miami*
9:55–10:35	Speaker Panel with Audience Participation
10:35–10:45	Break

CLOSING SESSION

10:45–11:45	Discussion: Research Gaps in Knowledge About Nutrition Interventions and Services for Older Adults in the Community Setting Moderator: Nancy Wellman, *Tufts University*
	Mary Ann Johnson *University of Georgia*
	Rebecca Costello *NIH Office of Dietary Supplements*
	Robert M. Russell *Tufts University*
	Judy Hannah *National Institute on Aging*
11:45 a.m.– 12:00 p.m.	Concluding Remarks and Closing Gordon L. Jensen, *Chair*

B

Moderator and Speaker Biographical Sketches

Connie W. Bales, Ph.D., R.D., is Professor of Medicine in the Division of Geriatrics, Department of Medicine, at the Duke School of Medicine and Senior Fellow in the Center for the Study of Aging and Human Development at Duke University Medical Center. She is also Associate Director for Education/Evaluation of the Geriatrics Research, Education and Clinical Center at the Durham VA Medical Center. Dr. Bales is a well-recognized expert in the field of nutrition and aging. Her research endeavors over the past two decades have focused on a variety of topics and she has published broadly on nutritional frailty, nutritional interventions for chronic diseases in aging, obesity in late life, and calorie restriction as a modifier of the aging process. She is the recipient of numerous awards, including the Grace Goldsmith Award and Max K. Horwitt Distinguished Lectureship. She currently serves the American Society for Nutrition as an Executive Member of the Medical Nutrition Council and is a past president of the American College of Nutrition. Dr. Bales edits the *Handbook of Clinical Nutrition in Aging* and the *Journal of Nutrition in Gerontology and Geriatrics*. Dr. Bales received her Ph.D. in 1981 at the University of Tennessee, Knoxville.

Enid A. Borden, M.S., is the President and Chief Executive Officer of the Meals On Wheels Association of America (MOWAA), the oldest and largest organization in the United States representing those who provide meal services to people in need. During her 19-year tenure at MOWAA, Ms. Borden has been responsible for the dramatic growth of the organization, leading it from a little-known trade group to a major national not-for-profit association and increasing its budget over tenfold. Her visionary leadership has not only made MOWAA the preeminent national organization dedicated to ending senior hunger in the United States but has also brought national attention to the long overlooked problem of senior hunger in America. Characterizing herself as a "missionary" in the cause of ending senior hunger in the United States, Enid Borden is frequently interviewed by major news media outlets and is often called upon by Congress, federal departments, and other not-for-profit organizations for expert advice and testimony. In addition to her position at MOWAA, Ms. Borden also serves as Chief Executive Officer of the Meals On Wheels Association of America Research Foundation. Prior to coming to MOWAA, Ms. Borden held several public affairs and policy positions in the public sector, including Deputy Commissioner for Policy and External Affairs at the Social Security Administration and Director of Public Affairs of the then Office of Human Development Services within the U.S. Department of Health and Human Services. She also has been a successful small business owner. Ms. Borden currently serves as an Advisory Board Member of the Sesame Street Food Insecurity Advisory Committee, on the American Society of Association Executive's (ASAE's) Key Philanthropic Organizations Committee, which she chaired in 2008 and 2009, and on the Board of Directors of the Visiting Nurse Associations of America. She has also been a member of the CEO Advisory Committee of ASAE, a member of the Nonprofit Advisory Board, and a Member of the Board of Trustees of Alfred University. Additionally, Ms. Borden has served on the faculty in the School of Graduate and Continuing Studies at Goucher College in Baltimore. Ms. Borden's work has earned her recognition in *Who's Who in the Media and Communications*. She earned her bachelor's degree from Alfred University, her master's degree from Adelphi University, and pursued study through the John F. Kennedy School of Government of Harvard University.

Eric A. Coleman, M.D., M.P.H., is Professor of Medicine and Head of the Division of Health Care Policy and Research at the University of Colorado at Denver. Dr. Coleman is the Director of the Care Transitions Program (www.caretransitions.org), which is aimed at improving quality and safety during times of care "hand-offs." He is also the Executive Director of the Practice Change Fellows Program (www.practicechangefellows.org), which is designed to build leadership capacity among health care professionals who are responsible for geriatric programs and service lines. Dr. Coleman bridges innovation and practice through (1) enhancing the role of patients and caregivers in improving the quality of their care transitions across acute and postacute settings, (2) measuring quality of care transitions from the perspective of patients and caregivers, (3) implementing system-level practice improvement interventions, and (4) using health information technology to promote safe and effective care transitions.

Charlene Compher, Ph.D., R.D., CNSC, LDN, FADA, is an Associate Professor of Nutrition Science at the University of Pennsylvania School of Nursing. She also is an advanced practice dietitian at the Hospital of the University of Pennsylvania, one of the top 10 hospitals in the United States. Dr. Compher is a highly regarded clinical researcher, clinician, and editor, whose research has focused on conditions with high nutritional risk, including severe gastrointestinal disease, the elderly, and obesity. Dr. Compher impacts practice from local to international levels by developing evidence-based clinical guidelines for nutrition support practice.

Rebecca Costello, Ph.D., recently retired from the National Institutes of Health (NIH) Office of Dietary Supplements (ODS) as Director of Grants and Extramural Activities, a position which she held for 6 years. Prior to that she was ODS Deputy Director from January 1999 to April 2006 and Acting Director from January 1999 to October 1999. Dr. Costello participated in the development of the ODS Strategic Plan and is charged with implementing the plan's goals and objectives by organizing workshops and conferences on dietary supplements, conducting scientific reviews to identify gaps in scientific knowledge, and initiating and coordinating research efforts among NIH Institutes and other federal agencies. As Director of Grants and Extramural Activities she encouraged partnerships with other NIH Institutes and Centers to facilitate funding of grants that are of high relevance to the ODS mission and goals. Prior to her NIH appointment, Dr. Costello was with the Food and Nutrition Board of the National Academy of Sciences, serving as Project Director for the Committee on Military Nutrition Research. She received a B.S. and M.S. in biology from the American University and a Ph.D. in clinical nutrition from the University of Maryland at College Park. Dr. Costello is a member of the American Society of Nutrition, American Heart Association, and the Southern Society of Clinical Investigation. She is also a liaison member to the Nutrition Committee of the American Heart Association and an adjunct assistant professor in the Department of Military and Emergency Medicine of the Uniformed Services University of the Health Sciences in Bethesda, Maryland.

Lori Gerhard is the Director of the Office of Program Innovation and Demonstration for the U.S. Administration on Aging (AoA). The Office has responsibility for helping to transform AoA core programs through innovation grant programs. Prior to joining AoA, Ms. Gerhard served as Acting Secretary of the Pennsylvania Department of Aging and she also has experience as a state policy maker, nursing home administrator, consultant and educator. With more than 27 years of experience in developing and delivering long-term services and supports, Ms. Gerhard has extensive knowledge and experience in the development of state long-term service and support

systems including financing, regulatory, and general operations. She has a
B.S. degree from the Pennsylvania State University's Health Planning and
Administration program and is a graduate of the University of North Texas'
Certified Aging Specialist Program.

Judy Hannah, Ph.D., is Health Science Administrator in the Division of
Geriatrics and Clinical Gerontology at the National Institute on Aging.

James A. Hester, Ph.D., is the Acting Director of the Population Health
Models Group at the Innovation Center in the Centers for Medicare &
Medicaid Services (CMS), developing new care models and payment reform
initiatives designed to improve the health of communities and targeted
populations. Prior to joining CMS, he was the Director of the Health Care
Reform Commission for the Vermont state legislature. The commission was
charged with overseeing the implementation of a comprehensive package
of health reform legislation and recommending the long-term strategy to
ensure that all Vermonters have access to affordable, quality health care.
The delivery system reforms included a statewide enhanced medical home
program and the development of pilot community health systems based on
the ACO concept. Dr. Hester has 35 years' experience in the health care
field, and has held senior management positions with MVP Healthcare in
Vermont, ChoiceCare in Cincinnati, Pilgrim Health Care in Boston, and
Tufts Medical Center in Boston. He began his managed care career as Director of Applied Research for the Kaiser Permanente Medical Care Program
in Los Angeles, California. Dr. Hester earned his Ph.D. in urban studies,
and his M.S. and B.S. degrees in aeronautics and astronautics, all from
the Massachusetts Institute of Technology. He has a continuing interest in
health services research and teaching, and has held faculty appointments
at the University of Vermont, University of Cincinnati, Harvard School of
Public Health, and the University of Massachusetts. He has served on the
boards of Vermont Information Technology Leaders (VITL), the Vermont
Program for Quality Health Care, and UVM's College of Nursing and
Health Science.

Gordon L. Jensen, M.D., Ph.D., is head of the Department of Nutritional Sciences at the Pennsylvania State University and former Director and Professor
of Medicine at the Vanderbilt Center for Human Nutrition. Dr. Jensen's research interests have focused largely on geriatric nutrition concerns. A major
limitation in the identification of elders at nutritional risk has been the lack
of valid methodologies that have been tested in rigorous research studies with
well-defined outcome measures. His team has therefore emphasized the development and testing of nutrition screening and assessment tools in relation to
specific functional and health care resource outcomes for older persons. In

particular he has focused upon the impact of obesity on these outcomes. At present he serves as a member of the Institute of Medicine (IOM) Food and Nutrition Board (FNB) and the Food Forum. Dr. Jensen is a past president of the American Society for Parenteral and Enteral Nutrition. He is a past-chair of the Medical Nutrition Council of the American Society for Nutrition. He has served on advisory panels or work groups for the National Institutes of Health and the American Dietetic Association, and was a member of the IOM FNB Committee on Nutrition Services for Medicare Beneficiaries. Dr. Jensen received his Ph.D. in nutritional biochemistry from Cornell University and his medical degree from Cornell University Medical College.

Mary Ann Johnson, Ph.D., is the Bill and June Flatt Professor in Foods and Nutrition and is a Faculty of Gerontology in the Department of Foods and Nutrition, College of Family and Consumer Sciences, at the University of Georgia. Dr. Johnson's expertise in human aging is in longevity, health promotion, nutrition, vitamins, minerals, dietary supplements, and diabetes prevention and management and she is well known for translating scientific information about nutrition and health into practical advice for older adults and the agencies that serve them. She has been a subcontractor and nutrition services provider for the Northeast Georgia Area Agency on Aging since 1998 and a co-investigator of the NIH-funded Georgia Centenarian Study for more than 20 years. She is a technical consultant for the Georgia Division of Aging Services and a co-developer of *Live Well Age Well*, a website developed for older people and their families and caregivers (www.livewellagewell.info). Dr. Johnson is a member of the American Society of Nutrition (ASN), the American Dietetic Association, the Institute of Food Technologies, and the inaugural class of national spokespeople for ASN. She serves on the editorial board of *Journal of Nutrition in Gerontology and Geriatrics* and as the Secretary-Treasurer for the ASN Medical Nutrition Council. Dr. Johnson is a recipient of the 2008 Georgia Diabetes Coalition Research Award, the 2008 UGA College of Family and Consumer Sciences Outreach Award, and the 2010 Teacher of the Year in Foods and Nutrition, and was the first recipient of the Bill and June Flatt Professorship at the University of Georgia. She is the author or co-author of more than 120 peer-reviewed publications. Dr. Johnson received her doctorate in nutritional sciences from the University of Wisconsin–Madison.

Heather Keller, R.D., Ph.D., is a nutrition epidemiologist and dietitian. Her research expertise includes nutrition risk screening, assessment, and nutrition intervention for seniors in general and seniors with dementia in particular. Her research spans community and institutional sectors. She is a Professor in the Department of Family Relations and Applied Nutrition at the University of Guelph (Ontario, Canada) and a Research Scientist with the RBJ Schlegel-University of Waterloo Research Institute of Aging. As of January 2012, Dr. Keller is the Schlegel Research Chair in Nutrition and Aging at the University of Waterloo. Dr. Keller has published extensively in the area of nutrition and older adults. Her current research is focused on eating in dementia, social aspects of eating, weight loss, nutrition risk programs, and interventions. She is co-chair of the Canadian Malnutrition Task Force. In 2007 she received the Betty Havens Knowledge Translation Award from the Institute of Aging, CIHR. Dr. Keller engages in extensive community engaged scholarship and knowledge translation and exchange. Please see www.drheatherkeller.com for further details.

Neva Kirk-Sanchez, Ph.D., PT, is an Associate Professor of Clinical Physical Therapy at the University of Miami Miller School of Medicine. She has clinical experience in geriatric rehabilitation and health promotion and wellness in older populations. She also has a particular interest in the management of childhood and adult obesity. Her research interests include the impact of physical activity on chronic disease management. She has spoken widely on this topic in both community setting and to health care workers. She has a particular interest in the areas of type 2 diabetes, Alzheimer's disease, and other cognitive impairments, and physical activity in normal aging. She is currently engaged in a clinical trial of the effects of physical exercise versus cognitive exercise for people with mild cognitive impairment. Dr. Kirk-Sanchez has published articles in *Physical Therapy*; the *Journal of Geriatric Physical Therapy*; the *Journal of Physical Therapy Policy, Administration and Leadership*; and the *American Journal of Public Health*. She has also co-authored a guidebook for physical activity and nutrition education for the older adult with the National Resource Center for Nutrition, Physical Activity, and Aging funded by the Administration on Aging, and authored a book chapter on the impact of exercise on psychiatric disorders and diabetes mellitus.

Elizabeth B. Landon, R.D., L.D., is Vice President, Community Services for CareLink, the Central Arkansas Area Agency on Aging, Inc. Programs and services under her management include Client Representation, Family Caregiver, Medicare Part D Assistance, Volunteer Ombudsman, State Older Worker, Senior Companion, Congregate Meals, Meals On Wheels, and Adult Day Care. Ms. Landon is past president (1994–1996) of the Meals On Wheels Association of America (MOWAA) and also served as vice president, treasurer, and regional representative for MOWAA. She is past chair and a current member of the Board of Directors of the MOWAA Research Foundation and a former member of the Blue Ribbon Advisory Council (1991–1995) for the Nutrition Screening Initiative which was composed of health, medical, and aging professionals working together to reach agreement on risk factors affecting the health of older Americans. Ms. Landon holds a B.S. degree in general science from the University of Central Arkansas, attended the University of Arkansas in the master degree program in foods and nutrition, and completed an administrative/clinical dietetic internship at the University of Arkansas for Medical Sciences/ Veterans Administration in Little Rock, Arkansas.

Kathryn Larin is an Assistant Director with the Government Accountability Office (GAO) Education, Workforce, and Income Security team, where she oversees work on a broad range of issues affecting low-income workers, families, and children. She has conducted evaluations of a number of federal programs in the areas of economic and nutrition assistance, workforce development, social services, and education. Prior to coming to GAO, Ms. Larin served as a research analyst with the Center on Budget and Policy Priorities' Income Security Division. She also worked with the Department of Education's Planning and Evaluation Service and with the U.S. Senate Appropriations Committee. Ms. Larin graduated from Swarthmore College with a B.A. in economics and received a master's in public affairs from Princeton University's Woodrow Wilson School.

Jean Lloyd, M.S., has served as the National Nutritionist for the U.S. Administration on Aging in Washington, DC, since 1992. The U.S. Administration on Aging, within the Department of Health and Human Services, administers the Older Americans Act (OAA), which establishes a comprehensive and coordinated system of community-based supportive and nutrition services to older people, including congregate and home-delivered nutrition services programs. During her time with the agency, she has been responsible and provided input for the nutrition related functions of policy, budget, legislation, and regulation; program development and implementation; training and technical assistance; advocacy; evaluation; and research, demonstration, and training grants. She also represents the agency as a member of the Dietary Reference Intake Steering Committee.

Julie L. Locher, Ph.D., M.S.P.H., is an Associate Professor in the Departments of Medicine and Health Care Organization and Policy at the University of Alabama at Birmingham (UAB). She also serves as Director of the Public Policy and Aging Program at UAB, jointly sponsored by the Center for Aging and the Lister Hill Center for Health Policy. She is a Medical Sociologist and Health Services Researcher. Dr. Locher's research has been supported consistently by the National Institute on Aging for the past decade. Her primary area of research focuses on social and environmental factors, including community and health care practices and policies that affect eating behaviors and nutrition-related health outcomes in older adults.

Most of this work has been observational, but is now turning toward interventional research and health services research utilizing large databases. A second and related area of interest focuses on examining practices and policies that affect the overall well-being of older adults and cancer patients and survivors, and identifying ways to best deliver quality care and services, especially that related to nutritional well-being, to these populations over the long term.

Robert H. Miller, Ph.D., is Divisional Vice President of Global Research and Development and Scientific Affairs at Abbott Nutrition. He joined Abbott in 1987 and has held several management positions in R&D and Technology Assessment. Dr. Miller left Abbott to join Battelle Memorial Institute as Director of Biotechnology in 2001. He is a member of the Abbott Scientific Governing Board. Dr. Miller earned his bachelor's degree in biochemistry from the University of Minnesota and his Ph.D. in nutritional science from the University of Wisconsin–Madison followed by a staff fellowship at NIH.

Bobbie L. Morris works at the Alabama Department of Senior Services in Montgomery, Alabama. She has over 30 years experience in food, nutrition and the continuum of care for older adults. She has worked in care settings that include hospital, home health, nursing home, assisted living and now with the Alabama Elderly Nutrition Program. She assists in monitoring the state meal contract with Valley Food Service by on-site visits to the 350 senior centers and 6 commissaries in the state. Ms. Morris regularly goes into the senior centers where congregate meals are served, and homes of the recipients of door-to-door meal deliveries. She has seen and heard from participants and staff who share about the advantages of receiving prepared meals in congregate settings and at home. In addition to monitoring, she also provides nutrition and food safety education to participants, senior center managers, and nutrition coordinators throughout the state. Ms. Morris holds a B.S. degree from the University of Alabama and is a registered, licensed dietitian and a Certified ServSafe instructor.

Douglas Paddon-Jones, Ph.D., is Associate Professor in the Department of Physical Therapy, with a joint appointment in the Department of Internal Medicine, Division of Endocrinology. He is the General Clinical Research Center Director of Exercise Studies, and a Fellow of the University of Texas Medical Branch (UTMB) Sealy Center on Aging at UTMB and vice-chair of UTMB's Institutional Review Board. Dr. Paddon-Jones' research focuses on mechanisms contributing to skeletal muscle protein synthesis and breakdown and identification of interventions to counteract muscle loss in healthy and clinical populations. He has conducted several

National Institutes of Health and NASA/National Space Biomedical Research Institute supported bed-rest studies, including studies investigating the effects of artificial gravity and amino acid supplementation on muscle protein metabolism. Dr. Paddon-Jones has undergraduate degrees in medical imaging and physiology from the Queensland Institute of Technology and the University of Queensland, a master's degree in exercise physiology from Ball State University, and a Ph.D. in human movement studies from the University of Queensland. He was the 2006 recipient of the Vernon R. Young International Award for Amino Acid Research.

Robert M. Russell, M.D., is Professor Emeritus of Medicine and Nutrition at Tufts University. Dr Russell has served on many national and international advisory boards including the USDA Human Investigation Committee (Chairman), the FDA, the US Pharmacopoeia Convention, the National Institutes of Health, the World Health Organization, UNICEF, and the American Board of Internal Medicine. He has worked on international nutrition programs in several countries including Vietnam, Iran, Iraq, Guatemala, China, and the Philippines. Dr. Russell is a member of numerous professional societies, on the editorial boards of five professional journals, a past president of the American Society for Clinical Nutrition, and a former member of the Board of Directors of the American College of Nutrition. He is the immediate Past President of the American Society for Nutrition. Dr. Russell co-edited the last three editions of *Present Knowledge in Nutrition* and until recently was the Editor-in-Chief of *Nutrition Reviews*. He is staff physician emeritus at the Tufts University Medical Center. Dr. Russell served as a member of the IOM's Panels on Folate, Other B Vitamins, and Choline, and as chair of the Panel on Micronutrients. He is former chair of the Food and Nutrition Board and a fellow of the American Society for Nutrition. Dr Russell presently serves as a specialist-advisor to the National Institutes of Health and its BOND project in the United States, as a board member of the Nestle and Fetzer Foundations, and is on the board of trustees of the US Pharmacopeia. He has received numerous national and international awards for his research on retinoids and carotenoids, and has authored over 300 scientific papers and 5 books.

Nadine R. Sahyoun, Ph.D., R.D., is Associate Professor of Nutritional Epidemiology at the Department of Nutrition and Food Science, University of Maryland in College Park. Her area of work is on the impact of lifestyle factors and physical functioning on dietary intake and nutritional status of older adults, and consequently on chronic disease and mortality. Previously, Dr. Sahyoun served as a Nutritionist at the USDA Center for Nutrition Policy and Promotion in Washington, DC, and as a Senior Staff Fellow for the Office of Analysis, Epidemiology and Health Promotion for the National Center for Health Statistics in Hyattsville, Maryland. She has also served as Acting Director of the Nutrition Services Department at the Jean Mayer USDA Human Nutrition Research Center on Aging at Tufts University, and as Assistant Director of the Office of Nutrition of the Massachusetts Department of Public Health. Dr. Sahyoun earned her B.A. from the University of Massachusetts, Boston, and her M.S. in nutrition from the University of Iowa. She received her Ph.D. in nutrition from the Friedman School of Nutrition Science and Policy, at Tufts University and served as a postdoctoral research fellow with the Association for Teachers in Preventive Medicine Office of Analysis, Epidemiology and Health Promotion at the National Center for Health Statistics in Hyattsville, Maryland.

Daniel J. Schoeps is the Director, Purchased Long-Term Care Group in the Office of Geriatrics & Extended Care, U.S. Department of Veterans Affairs. He is the National Program Officer for all long-term care services purchased by VA. He was the senior staffer and principal writer of "VA Long-Term Care at the Crossroads," a blueprint for VA's expansion of home- and community-based services. Mr. Schoeps was awarded the Hubert H. Humphrey Award for Service to America by the Secretary for Health and Human Services, and the Federal Public Service Award by the National PACE Association.

Joseph R. Sharkey, Ph.D., M.P.H., R.D., is a Professor in the Department of Social and Behavioral Health, School of Rural Public Health (SRPH) at The Texas A&M Health Sciences Center in College Station, Texas; Director of the Texas Healthy Aging Research Network Collaborating Center; Director of the Texas Nutrition and Obesity Policy Research and Evaluation Network Collaborating Center; and Director of the Program for Research in Nutrition and Health Disparities at SRPH. Dr. Sharkey is currently Principal Investigator on three interdisciplinary research programs that examine complex, place-based factors that may either enable or constrain rural and underserved families from achieving and maintaining good nutritional health: (1) "Behavioral and Environmental Influence on Obesity: Rural Context & Race/Ethnicity," which is a 5-year project funded as part of a new NIH/NCMHD-funded Program for Rural and Minority Health Disparities Research at SRPH; (2) Core Research Program ("Working with Rural and Underserved Communities to Promote a Healthy Food Environment") within the SRPH Center for Community Health Development, a Prevention Research Center; and (3) "Influence of Mobile Food Vendors on Food and Beverage Choices of Low-Income Mexican American Children in Texas *Colonias*," funded by the Robert Wood Johnson Healthy Eating Research Program. He also serves as Chair of the SB 343 Healthy Food Advisory Committee, Texas Health and Human Services Commission and Texas Department of Agriculture. Dr. Sharkey's main areas of interest include food access and food choice in rural and underserved areas, measurement of household and neighborhood food environments, and nutritional and functional assessment. He received his M.P.H. and Ph.D. from the Department of Nutrition at the University of North Carolina at Chapel Hill School of Public Health.

Jennifer L. Troyer, Ph.D., is Associate Professor and Chair of the Department of Economics at the University of North Carolina at Charlotte, where she also holds an Adjunct Associate Professor appointment in the Department of Public Health Sciences. Dr. Troyer has published extensively in the area of health economics and the economics of aging. Her work includes three papers using data from a multiyear study funded by the Administration on Aging to examine the cost effectiveness of medical nutrition therapy, a form of intensive, specialized nutrition education, and of therapeutically designed meals provided to older adults diagnosed with hyperlipidemia and/or hypertension.

Katherine L. Tucker, Ph.D., is Professor and Chair, Department of Health Sciences, at Northeastern University. Previously she was Senior Scientist and Director of the Dietary Assessment and Epidemiology Research Program at the USDA Human Nutrition Research Center on Aging at Tufts University, and Professor and Director of the Nutritional Epidemiology Program for the Gerald J. and Dorothy R. Friedman School of Nutrition Science and Policy at Tufts University, where she holds an adjunct appointment. Her research interests include diet and health, nutrition in older adults, dietary methodology, nutritional status of high-risk populations, and nutritional epidemiology. She previously served on the IOM Committee on the Implications of Dioxin in the Food Supply and the IOM Committee to Review Child and Adult Care Food Program Meal Requirements. Dr. Tucker is an Associate Editor for the *Journal of Nutrition* and is currently the chair of the Nutritional Sciences Council of the American Society for Nutrition. In addition, she is a member of the American Society for Bone and Mineral Research and the Gerontological Society of America. Dr. Tucker received her B.Sc. in nutritional sciences from the University of Connecticut and her Ph.D. in nutrition sciences from Cornell University.

Elena Volpi, M.D., Ph.D., is a professor of Internal Medicine-Geriatrics and Neuroscience and Cell Biology at the University of Texas Medical Branch (UTMB), the director of the UTMB Claude D. Pepper Older Americans Independence Center (OAIC), and the Associate Director of the Institute for Translational Sciences-CTSA. She was nominated a Brookdale National Fellow in the year 2000 and is the principal investigator of the OAIC and two R01 grants, all funded by the NIA. She has published extensively in peer-reviewed journals in the area of muscle function, nutrition, and metabolism in older adults. Her research program is centered on understanding the mechanisms responsible for the age-related sarcopenia, and preventing sarcopenia, frailty, and functional dependence in older adults.

Edwin L. Walker, J.D., is Deputy Assistant Secretary for Program Operations with the AoA within the U.S. Department of Health and Human Services. He serves as the chief career official for the federal agency responsible for advocating on behalf of older Americans. In this capacity, he guides and promotes the development of home and community-based long-term care programs, policies and services designed to afford older people and their caregivers the ability to age with dignity and independence and to have a broad array of options available for an enhanced quality of life. This includes the promotion and implementation of evidence-based prevention interventions proven effective in avoiding or delaying the onset of chronic disease and illness. A strong and experienced advocate for older persons, he has served as the primary liaison with Congress on legislation related to aging services and programs. For more than 25 years, he has been characterized as a consummate professional civil servant who can be relied upon to represent the best interests of our nation's senior citizens. Prior to joining the AoA, Mr. Walker served as the Director of the Missouri Division of Aging, responsible for administering a comprehensive set of human service programs for older persons and adults with disabilities. He received a J.D. from the University of Missouri-Columbia School of Law and a B.A. in mass media arts from Hampton University.

Elizabeth A. Walker, Ph.D., R.N., is a Professor of Medicine and Professor of Epidemiology & Population Health, and the director of the Prevention and Control Core for the NIH-funded Diabetes Research Center (DRC) at the Albert Einstein College of Medicine, Bronx, New York. Dr. Walker is principal investigator of a large NIH-funded behavioral intervention study in minority diabetes populations, using telephonic interventions in Spanish and English to promote medication adherence and other self-management behaviors. She is also PI of a research-capacity-building NIH grant with South Bronx community health centers. Since 1995, she has been a behavioral scientist and co-investigator for the multicenter Diabetes Prevention Program (DPP) and Outcomes Study, and she co-chairs the DPP Medication Adherence Committee. Through the Prevention and Control Core of the DRC she provides or facilitates various intervention and evaluation services to multiple health disparities projects in the community. Elizabeth is a diabetes nurse specialist and has been a certified diabetes educator (CDE) since 1986. In 2000, she served as the national President, Health

Care & Education, of the American Diabetes Association. She is a Fellow of the American Association of Diabetes Educators (FAADE). Dr. Walker is a behavioral scientist with the Einstein Diabetes Global Health team for Uganda in East Africa.

Nancy S. Wellman, Ph.D., is an affiliated faculty member at Tufts University's Friedman School of Nutrition Science and Policy. She recently retired as the Professor of Dietetics and Nutrition in the School of Public Health at Florida International University, the public research university in Miami. She is the former director of the National Resource Center on Nutrition, Physical Activity and Aging. Dr. Wellman is a past President of the American Dietetic Association and has been a member of committees for the National Academy of Sciences and the Institute of Medicine. She currently serves as Chair of the Board of Directors for the International Food Information Council Foundation, is a member of the American Society for Nutrition (ASN) Public Information Committee and is an ASN national spokesperson.

James P. Ziliak, Ph.D., holds the Carol Martin Gatton Endowed Chair in Microeconomics in the Department of Economics and is Founding Director of the Center for Poverty Research at the University of Kentucky. He served as assistant and associate professor of economics at the University of Oregon, and has held visiting positions at the Brookings Institution, University College London, University of Michigan, and University of Wisconsin. His research expertise is in the areas of labor economics, poverty, food insecurity, and tax and transfer policy. Recent projects include an examination of the causes and consequences of hunger among older Americans; a study of trends in earnings and income volatility in the United States; the effects of welfare reform on earnings of single mothers; regional wage differentials across the earnings distribution; and the geographic distribution of poverty under alternative poverty measures. He is editor of the books *Welfare Reform and its Long Term Consequences for America's Poor* published by Cambridge University Press (2009) and *Appalachian Legacy: Economic Opportunity after the War on Poverty* published by Brookings Institution Press (2012).

C

Workshop Attendees

Dawn Alley
University of Maryland
Washington, DC

Catherine Anderton
Unity Healthcare Organization
Washington, DC

Victoria Bailey-Makinde
Washington, DC

Lura Barber
National Council on Aging
Washington, DC

Judy Berger
Jefferson Area Board for Aging
Charlottesville, VA

Dondeena Bradley
PepsiCo
Purchase, NY

Shirley Bridgewater
Crater District Area Agency on
    Aging
Petersburg, VA

Linda Bruce
Washington, DC

David Buys
University of Alabama at
    Birmingham
Birmingham, AL

Mark Byron
USDA
Alexandria, VA

Sandy Campbell
Meals On Wheels Research
    Foundation
Alexandria, VA

Yumi Chiba
Philadelphia, PA

Kristine Choe
Fairfax County Government
Oak Hill, VA

Rose Clifford
IONA
Washington, DC

Nancy L. Cohen
University of Massachusetts
Amherst, MA

Kirsten Colello
Library of Congress
Washington, DC

David Dennis
Abbott Nutrition
Columbus, OH

Rose Ann DiMaria-Ghalili
Drexel University
Philadelphia, PA

Shannon Dodd
Fairfax County Government
Fairfax, VA

Shannon Donahue
National Association of Nutrition
    and Aging Services Programs
Washington, DC

Anne Dumas
Abbott Nutrition
Montreal, CAN

Anne Dunlop
Emory University
Atlanta, GA

Donna Dunston
Silver Spring, MD

Sarah Fisher
Washington, DC

Molly French
Potomac Health Consulting
Arlington, VA

Jackie Geralnick
Grocery Manufacturers Association
Washington, DC

Daniel Green
Rosslyn, VA

Teresa Green
National Consumers League
Washington, DC

Marcia Greenblum
Egg Nutrition Center
Kensington, MD

Carolyn Gugger
General Mills
Minneapolis, MN

Magda Hageman-Apol
Meals On Wheels Association of
    America
Alexandria, VA

Robert Herbolsheimer
Meals On Wheels Association of
    America
Alexandria, VA

Amy Herring
USDA
Washington, DC

Harriet Herry
Mitchellville, MD

Adele Hite
University of North Carolina
Durham, NC

Karen Jackson Holzhauer
Area Agency on Aging
Southfield, MI

Kelly Horton
National Council on Aging
Washington, DC

Margaret Ingraham
Meals On Wheels Association of
    America
Alexandria, VA

Erika Kelly
Meals On Wheels Association of
    America
Alexandria, VA

Karin Kolsky
National Institutes of Health
Bethesda, MD

Kathryn Larin
Government Accountability Office
Washington, DC

Joe Layton
Raleigh, NC

James Lee
University of District of Columbia
Washington, DC

Gladys Mason
Petersburg, VA

Patricia Matthews
Department of Health and Senior
    Services
Trenton, NJ

Holly McPeak
Department of Health and Senior
    Services
Rockville, MD

Michelle Miller
Fairfax County Government
Fairfax, VA

Amber Mills
Washington, DC

Evelyn Minor
Washington, DC

Debra Mobley
Loudoun County Government
Leesburg, VA

Lillie Monroe-Lord
University of the District of
    Columbia
Washington, DC

Amy Nagy
Fairfax County Government
Fairfax, VA

Danielle Nelson
Administration on Aging
Washington, DC

Linda Netterville
Meals On Wheels Association of
    America
Alexandria, VA

Melissa O'Connor
Fairfax County Government
Fairfax, VA

Gordon O'Keefe
Burke, VA

Chitua Okoh
Bowie, MD

Eleese Onami
Providence Hospital
Washington, DC

Rex O'Rourke
National Association of States
    United for Aging and
    Disabilities
Washington, DC

Carol O'Shaughnessy
National Health Policy Forum
Washington, DC

Katie Pahner
Health Policy Source
Washington, DC

Kourtney Parman
Washington, DC

Melissa Pember
Washington, DC

Mary Penet
Feed More
Richmond, VA

Sonia Pessoa
Vida Senior Centers
Washington, DC

Melanie Polk
Montgomery County Government
Rockville, MD

Mary Pat Raimondi
Eat Right
Washington, DC

Karen Regan
National Institute of Health
Bethesda, MD

Lynn Reid
Loudoun County Government
Leesburg, VA

Edgar Rivas
University Park, MD

Sarah Roholt
Raleigh, NC

David Sadowski
Crater District Area Agency on
    Aging
Petersburg, VA

Mallory Schindler
American Academy of Nursing
Washington, DC

Malini Sekhar
Meals On Wheels Research
    Foundation
Alexandria, VA

Judy Simon
Maryland Department of Aging
Baltimore, MD

Danfeng Song
Food and Drug Administration
College Park, MD

Kathryn Strong
Leesburg, VA

Katherine Tallmadge
Washington, DC

Amy Tan
H2F Advisory Services
Reston, VA

Jason Thrush
Abbott Nutrition
Columbus, OH

Jane Tilly
Administration on Aging
Washington, DC

Cheryl Toner
Document Communication
    Technologies
Fairfax, VA

Anisa Tootla
AARP
Washington, DC

Lauren Trocchio
Washington, DC

Lisa Troy
Institute of Medicine
Washington, DC

Laurie Tucker
Well Styles Consulting
Bethesda, MD

Allison Valle
Seabury Resources
Washington, DC

Charlene Ward
New Carrollton, MD

Susan Welsh
Harford County Office on Aging
Bel Air, MD

Tara West
Fairfax County Government
Fairfax, VA

Tiffany Westover-Kernan
Corporate Voices
Alexandria, VA

Debra Williams
Loudoun County Government
Leesburg, VA

Violet Woo
HHS
Rockville, MD

Tiffanie Yates
Washington, DC, Government
Washington, DC

Ellen Young
Lake Country Area Agency on
    Aging
Manson, NC

D

Abbreviations and Acronyms

ACO	Accountable Care Organization
ADLs	activities of daily living
AI	Adequate Intake
AoA	Administration on Aging
BMI	body mass index
CACFP	Child and Adult Care Food Program
CBO	community-based organization
CCTP	Community Based Care Transition Program
CDSMP	Chronic Disease Self-Management Program, Stanford University
CFSM	Core Food Security Module
CMS	Centers for Medicare & Medicaid Services
CN	congregate nutrition services
CPS	Current Population Survey
CSFP	Commodity Supplemental Food Program
CTI	Care Transitions Intervention®
DASH	Dietary Approach to Stop Hypertension
DGA	*Dietary Guidelines for Americans*
DGAC	Dietary Guidelines Advisory Committee
DOT	Department of Transportation

DPP	Diabetes Prevention Program
DRI	Dietary Reference Intake
EAR	Estimated Average Requirement
FMS	financial management services
FNB	Food and Nutrition Board, Institute of Medicine, The National Academies
FY	fiscal year
GAO	Government Accountability Office
HDN	home-delivered nutrition services
HHS	Department of Health and Human Services
HUP	Hospital of the University of Pennsylvania
IOM	Institute of Medicine, The National Academies
MNT	medical nutrition therapy
MOWAA	Meals On Wheels Association of America
NH	nursing home
NHANES	National Health and Nutrition Examination Survey
NIA	National Institute on Aging
NIH	National Institutes of Health
OAA	Older Americans Act
P.L.	public law
QALY	quality-adjusted life year
QIO	Quality Improvement Organization
RD	registered dietitian
RDA	Recommended Daily Allowance
SNAP	Supplemental Nutrition Assistance Program
SOW	statement of work
TEFAP	The Emergency Food Assistance Program
USDA	U.S. Department of Agriculture

VA	Veterans Administration
VD-HCBS	Veterans Directed Home- and Community-Based Services
VHA	Veterans Health Administration
WIC	Special Supplemental Nutrition Program for Women, Infants, and Children